/EAST.GV461.U531979>C1/

DISCARD

W9-CAR-345

East GV 461 .U53 1979
United States Gymnastics
 Safety Association.
Gymnastics safety manual :

52165

Oakton Community College
Morton Grove, Illinois

OAKTON COMMUNITY COLLEGE LIBRARY
EAST GV461 U531979   C001
GYMNASTICS SAFETY MANUAL 2D

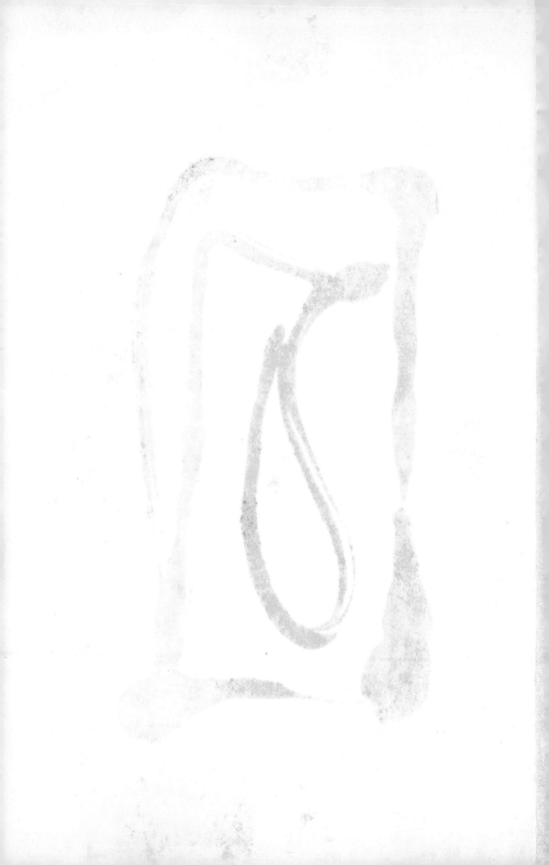

Gymnastics Safety Manual

Second Edition

DISCARD

Contributors to Text

Norman Barnes / Robert J. Bevenour / Cap Caudill
Roy Davis / Thomas L. Dunn, Jr. / Stormy Eaton
David A. Feigley / Larry Fie / A. B. Frederick
Jay Geist / Abie Grossfeld / Jeff T. Hennessy / Eric Hughes /
Loyd J. Huval / Edmund Isabelle / Mike Jacki
Alexander Kalenak, M.D. / Rich Kenney / Edgar M. Knepper
Hayes Kruger / Carole Liedtke / David J. Lindstrom
Newton C. Loken / Ruth Ann McBride / Ron Manara
Rodi Nikitins / Gary R. Seibert / Karl K. Schwenzfeier
Robert Stout / William G. Strauss / George Szypula
Donald R. Tonry / Zahir Toby Towson / Betty van der Smissen, J.D.
Gregor Weiss / Margie Weiss / Eugene Wettstone
Robert J. Willoughby

Gymnastics Safety Manual, Second Edition

The Official Manual
of the
United States Gymnastics Safety Association

Eugene Wettstone, Editor

with the assistance of Raleigh DeGeer Amyx,
Robert J. Bevenour, Larry Fie,
A. B. Frederick, Betty van der Smissen

OAKTON COMMUNITY COLLEGE
7900 NORTH NAGLE
MORTON GROVE, IL 60058

52165

The Pennsylvania State University Press
University Park and London

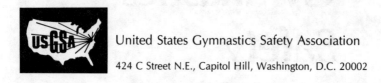

United States Gymnastics Safety Association

424 C Street N.E., Capitol Hill, Washington, D.C. 20002

President and Executive Director: Raleigh DeGeer Amyx

Board of Directors: Dave Bresnahan
Cap Caudill
Kathy Corrigan Ekas
J.B. Ford
Gerald George
Tom Heineike
Chris W. Kentera
Ruth Ann McBride
Eugene Wettstone

Second Edition, October 1979

cloth ISBN 0-271-00242-5
paper ISBN 0-271-00244-1
LC 79-65860

Copyright © 1979 The Pennsylvania State University
All rights reserved

Designed by Glenn Ruby
Drawings in text by C.K. Bingham — except those in Chapter 10, which are from Hennessey, Jeff T., *Trampolining*, Brown Physical Education Activities Series, 1968, Wm. C. Brown Company Publishers, Dubuque, Iowa.

Printed in the United States of America

Foreword

This manual by the United States Gymnastics Safety Association is one of the first covering the discipline necessary in a specific sport—in the tradition of the Red Cross Swimming and Water Safety Manuals. I compliment the board members and the coaches for their foresight in pressing forward with this very thoughtful teaching manual. Such a publication will be of particular value to the many new teachers emerging from our teacher preparation institutions, not just for the sake of appreciating the risk involved in every vigorous activity but even more from the standpoint of developing sound methods of teaching the skills in the sport of gymnastics.

The chapters contributed demonstrate outstanding authoritativeness when one examines the records and the backgrounds of their authors. I know most of them and have seen most of them in action, including Dr. Betty van der Smissen, professor in recreation and law; the four Olympic coaches; the six Olympians; the dozen national gymnastic champions; the ten authors of outstanding textbooks; and Dr. Alexander Kalenak, Hershey Medical Center, an orthopedic surgeon of great renown. The reader must feel honored to be able to absorb this wealth of information by people who have such credentials and who have done this work so that the sport may continue to grow in a healthier and safer climate.

The national program of physical fitness and sports stresses gymnastics as one of the priority activities. The President's Council on Physical Fitness and Sports (PCPFS) and its staff are advocates of programs which contain some element of risk. A sports program in which one cannot fail is a program in which one cannot succeed. The PCPFS feels that a sport that does not have some element of risk is a sport that contributes nothing. Unfortunately, many of our youth grow to adulthood without participating in anything which involves sweat, discomfort, or effort. Erroneously, some teachers and leaders have placed the highest premium on "fun" as the major objective of physical education and sports.

Gymnastics provides the real satisfaction of achievement and the complementary outcome of good physical condition. In the interest of the nation's health, we need vigorous activities throughout our lives. Unfortunately, cutbacks in physical education and sports and over-protection of youth have resulted in losses in the physical fitness of our youth. Gymnastics is one of the four survival activities in physical education, along with combative sports, swimming, and physical conditioning. The national goal of preventive medicine is to keep people out of the doctor's office.

No matter what safety measures are applied, there will always be some elements of risk and some accidents sometimes. The environment is not going to adjust to an individual. Individuals have to prepare themselves to meet the emergencies in life . . . this is the "guts" in our sports program.

Even more than physical preparedness, sports develop an attitude . . . God Bless the Coaches and Athletic Teachers of this Nation.

C. Carson Conrad

Executive Director
President's Council on Physical Fitness and Sports

Preface

The aim of this manual is to raise the level of safety in those recreational and athletic activities generally described as gymnastics: tumbling and floor exercises; vaulting over gym horses; and skills performed on pommel horses, still rings, balance beams, horizontal bars, even or uneven parallel bars, and the trampoline. The value of gymnastics for physical education, sport, and health has been emphasized by the President's Council on Physical Fitness and Sports, as its executive director states in his foreword.

Thanks to gymnastics' contagious appeal — conveyed both by individual enthusiasm and by media coverage of gymnastic events including those of the Olympic Games — gymnastics is growing rapidly in popularity. Such growth naturally brings both opportunities and challenges to persons who sponsor or direct gymnastic activities — or who are preparing to do so. The prime challenge is to develop and maintain the highest possible level of safety in an area of activity where a high degree of vigorous involvement and dedicated practice is demanded — where, indeed, these qualities are of the essence.

This manual covers those factors that must be considered in a conscientious effort to assure a safe gymnastic environment, safely prepared gymnasts, and safe gymnastic supervision and instruction. Since accidents and emergencies are unavoidable in human affairs, possible medical and legal consequences are explored. Preparation and care measures are presented honestly, not as guarantees against injuries and potential lawsuits but as the best form of insurance.

This manual is directed to all persons engaged in, or preparing for, the teaching or supervision of gymnastics programs. Such programs may be in public or private schools, colleges, or universities; fraternal, social, or youth organizations; and private clubs or camps. The directly concerned persons may be specialists in gymnastics instruction; physical education teachers and administrators with some responsibility for gymnastics; gymnastics coaches, assistant coaches, and trainers — or they may be students preparing for any of these roles. For all these, the USGSA Teacher Certification Program described in Chapter 13 (for which this book is the text) is recommended. For the many others with a less direct responsibility — school and college administrators and trustees, club officers and directors, and affiliated medical and legal personnel — the *Gymnastics Safety Manual* is recommended as invaluable background information.

Eugene Wettstone

Message from USGSA President

In the process of preparing for the publication of the second edition of the *Gymnastics Safety Manual* it occurs to me that readers would be interested in a brief synopsis of our Association's objectives and goals. These objectives and goals are being realized.

From the outset, our prime objective was the development of a stringent Gymnastics Safety Certification Program for professionals in gymnastics. Goals of this program are to

- Help reduce accidents and their severity
- Provide an independent professional recognition system for those who are actually qualified to instruct safely
- Prove to school administrators that gymnastics has a positive safety program
- Put our coaches in a legally defensible position in the event of an unfortunate accident
- Make gymnastics the first organized sport to establish Safety Certification of coaches for the protection of athletes

The need is obvious, and we are pleased to have had strong support from the American National Red Cross and the President's Council on Physical Fitness and Sports. In the first eighteen months since the inception of USGSA Certification on January 1, 1978 more than 2,000 of our nation's gymnastics coaches have become USGSA Safety Certified. And our membership now exceeds 3,500 universities, high schools, organizations such as the YMCA or YWCA, and individual gymnastics coaches or teachers.

It was a particular pleasure to have had the first edition of the *Gymnastics Safety Manual* selected by the Association of American University Presses as one of the top 25 books, in design and production, published in 1977.

Raleigh DeGeer Amyx, *President and Executive Director*
United States Gymnastics Safety Association
424 C Street, N.E., Capitol Hill, Washington, D.C.
20002

Acknowledgments

A safety manual and teacher certification program have been major projects of the United States Gymnastics Safety Association since its formation on May 1, 1976. The roots of the USGSA go back to the 1975 United States Gymnastic Congress in Denver, when a group of concerned coaches, educators, club owners, and equipment manufacturers met to discuss safety aspects of the sport. Safety standards for the sport, long a concern of most people associated with gymnastics, seemed clearly a subject that needed implementation. Founders of the USGSA owe a special debt of gratitude to the President's Council on Physical Fitness and Sports, the Consumer Product Safety Commission, the American National Red Cross, and the Sporting Goods Manufacturers Association for early and continuing encouragement and help.

The first step toward setting standards was taken when a workbook called "Guidelines to Safety in Gymnastics" was compiled by a group of USGSA friends and supporters led by Cap Caudill and John Fiore. All lovers of gymnastics are indebted to these pioneers.

Soon afterward Gene Wettstone, a gymnastic educator and coach of world renown, agreed to edit the present manual and develop a certification program. He first enlisted the full cooperation of his fellow USGSA board members, then of his colleagues in the College of Health, Physical Education, and Recreation of The Pennsylvania State University, notably Robert J. Scannell and Betty van der Smissen. Next Gene got expert help from Dr. Alexander Kalenak of his University's Hershey Medical Center and David Lindstrom of the Health Center. Gene then lined up specialists throughout the country to draft portions of the text. With this progression going, Gene arranged for publication of the *Gymnastics Safety Manual* by The Pennsylvania State University Press. Chris Kentera, Press Director, assigned Editorial Director John Pickering to work with Gene on final editorial development, ably assisted by the Press's Robert Paradine, Glenn Ruby, and Janet Dietz and Pennsylvania artist C. K. Bingham. The Press staff deserves great credit for the thorough development of this manual and for accomplishing publication in record time. Words cannot adequately express our gratitude to Gene Wettstone, without whom this project could not have been accomplished so soon or so well.

Our contributing authors are appropriately recognized on a special page. What a superior effort they made! But there are others, and without their collaboration this book would have been difficult to complete. Special thanks go to Cap Caudill and Dave Feigley for their constant encouragement. We also are delighted to recognize the contributions of talent and time extended by George Nissen, Larry Fie, Mike Jacki, Bob Bevenour, C. Carson Conrad, Howard J. Bruns, Frank Bare, Rich Kenney, Gary Seibert, Edgar Knepper, Dick Kellor, Glenn Sundby, Bruce Frederick, and Ed Isabelle. Others who took part in the early planning of this manual were: Murray Anderson, Tom Darling, John Fiore, Bruno Klaus, Jon and Boots Culbertson, Jay Geist, Ron Manara, Tom Jones, Bill and Ginny Coco, Floy Barnard, Doug Alt, Hayes Kruger, Marty Faust, Fred Turoff, Barbara Thatcher, Dave Bresnahan, Wayne Young, Karen Shuckman, Janette Anderson, Roxanne Pierce, Bill Strauss, Fred Surgent, and Laureen Tkacik.

A host of others have given generously of their time and experience. Notable among these are J. B. Ford, Mike Schneider, Art Goettler, Larry Montgomery, John Liskey, Jeff Hennessy, Raleigh Wilson, Robert Morris, C.M. DuBois, Barbara Ryder, Mary Ellen Jacobson, Mike Bisk, Don Volz, Paul Bohrer, Dick Schnaars, Marilyn Schnaars, Paul Spadaro, Kenny Vinyard, Ted Pritchett, Brian Gallagher, Barbara Gallagher, Nick Akins, Robbin Pritchett, Becky Robinson, Jeff Appling, Carey Culbertson, Bob Darden, Michele Amyx, Allison Hyland, Craig Nidever, Darlene Dolbow, Mike Mascaro, Lacrisha Bailey, Harriett Ford, Bill Cameron, John Howe, Steve Labe, Arlyn Black, John E. Harvey, Hilda Amyx, Charles B. Clark, Donald B. Wilderroter, Bennie Faye La Farque, and Judi Avener.

I am privileged to present this manual to you on behalf of our USGSA members and directors. We dedicate it to all who are devoted to the health and physical fitness of our youth and to the ideal of a sound mind in a strong body with moral integrity.

Raleigh DeGeer Amyx, *President and Executive Director*
United States Gymnastics Safety Association
424 C Street N.E., Capitol Hill, Washington, D.C.
20002

Contents

1

Developing Safety Awareness

Safety measures are as important to gymnastics as skills. When training in a gymnastic skill is introduced, it must be accompanied by appropriate safety measures. The instructor or coach's traditional moral responsibility for the safety of gymnasts—or aspiring gymnasts—now has the force of law. Lawsuits have established the principle that the gymnastic instructor or coach must be a "Reasonable and prudent *professional*" (see Chapter 11, Legal Responsibility in the Gymnasium). This principle is particularly important when the instructor is developing new techniques or original skills and combinations of skills. As a courtroom lawyer has said, "What the coach calls innovation, the court may call negligence."

Responsibility for gymnastic safety has two sides: prevention and remediation. Remediation is of vital importance, since accidents are not totally avoidable in any human activity—especially an activity involving physical exertion and proficiency—so remediation is covered in Chapter 10, Medical Responsibility in the Gymnasium. Prevention, however, is of first importance in both logic and law.

Prevention of gymnastic mishaps has three aspects as reflected in the organization of this manual: first, proper layout, selection, use, care, and staffing of gymnastic apparatus; second, proper physical preparedness and warm-up of gymnasts; third, proper progression in the teaching of skills. Fundamental to all three responsibilities is the development of safety awareness through cultivation of an analytical approach.

An analytical approach can be cultivated most effectively by asking appropriate questions and noting the possible consequences of inappropriate answers. Following are three lists of analytical questions. Although these lists reflect the experience of experts, no checklists can be exhaustive—so every reader is urged to make additions.

Is the Environment Prepared for the Performance of the Skill?

1. Has the instructor prepared the gymnasium with proper matting and safe, secure equipment?
2. Is the protective equipment properly positioned?
3. Is the protective equipment appropriate to the level of difficulty and/or risk of the skill to be attempted?
4. Is the protective equipment sufficient for the weight of the gymnast and the force of a fall should it occur?
5. Is the apparatus properly adjusted for the gymnast?
6. Have measures been taken to prevent accidental collisions with others by identifying approach and landing areas in which performers have the right of way?

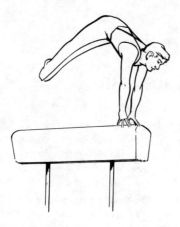

Is the Gymnast Prepared to Be Performing the Skill?

1. Does the gymnast have the physical abilities, strength, flexibility, and body awareness needed for the new skill?
2. Are the gymnast and instructor able to communicate clearly so that each understands his/her responsibilities during the learning of the skill?
3. Is the gymnast motivated to perform the skill?
4. Have the potential problems in the new skill learning experience been adequately identified to the satisfaction of both instructor and gymnast, and have measures been taken to eliminate or to minimize any risk?
5. Does the gymnast display or admit to any anxieties, doubts, or fears that could interfere with the safe performance of the skill?
6. Does the gymnast understand the mechanics of the skills and the sequence of necessary steps leading to mastery of the skills?
7. Has the gymnast attained sufficient mastery of the required subskills?

Is the Instructor Prepared to Teach the Skill?

1. Does the instructor have sufficient knowledge of the mechanics of the skill to be learned and the necessary subskills?
2. Is the instructor able to make specific adjustments in the learning sequence to accommodate the gymnast's needs whether real or imagined?
3. Is the instructor familiar with the level of mental preparedness of the gymnast and has the instructor determined if that preparedness is appropriate to the difficulty level of the skill?
4. Is the instructor capable of spotting the skill properly either by himself/herself or with qualified assistance?
5. In the event of special learner problems, is the instructor able to further divide the skill into smaller meaningful steps?

Responsibility

The chapters which follow will point out rather dramatically the many areas of responsibility of the gymnastic instructor/coach. Never before have we been so aware of the duties of a teacher to the youthful athletes in his care.

This section is here to remind the reader that listing rules and regulations is not enough. The responsibility of the instructor/coach is to carry out such precepts. It has been said that the competent and alert teacher does not need warnings and is safeguarded against errors. Unfortunately no teacher is constantly perfect, so the need for rules and reminders becomes imperative.

Even though gymnastic safety is everyone's responsibility, the instructor or coach must bear much of it, including the responsibility to see that others do their share: the parents, the doctor, the participant. Prevention and remediation are major responsibilities in a broad umbrella type program under which many other points must be included: the environment, the prescribed learning progression, and the physical preparedness of the participant. These are the areas where the instructor/coach bears much of the moral and legal responsibility. It is not enough to warn and inform; all concerned must have an appreciation and understanding of the risk in every vigorous activity. It can be said that the teacher has to be as much a psychologist and physiologist as a competent instructor of gymnastic skills. He has to have adequate knowledge of athletic training and essential first aid practices. In the event of a lawsuit arising from a gymnastic accident, it is no longer a sufficient defense to argue only an assumed risk on the part of the participant, because competent and vigilant supervision also is a reasonable expectation. Some instructors find class or individual progress reports a useful tool in supervision.

There is a great deal of responsibility to preparing the student properly in a safe environment. It behooves all readers of these chapters to be particularly alert and to make mental notes of those areas where the teacher/coach is responsible.

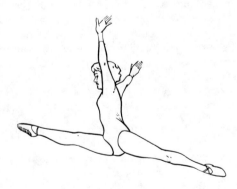

2

Gymnasium Facilities and Supervision

The physical facilities of a gymnasium must be planned with care for the human needs it is designed to serve—limited by the human resources available for supervision. A responsible professional will make sure his gymnasium has suitable space, apparatus, safety equipment, and supervisory staff for all the activities he plans and for all the participants he expects. Conversely, he will not start an activity until the physical facilities and supervisory arrangement assure safe participation by everyone concerned. Legally and morally, the gymnastic instructor or coach cannot defend himself by blaming someone else for a runway that is too narrow, a mat that is too thin, a bar that is too weak, or a spotter that is inattentive.

Layout, Safe Areas, and Staffing

The responsibility of a gymnastic instructor or coach in the planning of a gymnasium, whether it is being newly built or remodeled, is to assure the welfare and safety of *gymnasts,* regardless of the building's other uses. A gymnasium's utilization for basketball, volleyball, track and field events, and other sports—as well as non-athletic purposes such as meetings, plays, and concerts—should not be permitted to threaten gymnastic safety. Nor should accommodations for spectators or visitors of all ages interfere with properly supervised gymnastics.

Areas for gymnasts and their supervisors, for participants in concurrent activities such as running on an indoor track or trampolining, and for visitors and spectators must be separated by barriers or must be clearly marked. No one in a gymnasium should have any doubt as to where he or she belongs. Runways for gymnastic activities such as vaulting should be distinguished from walkways for non-working gymnasts, visitors, and spectators. Lobbies, grandstands or bleachers, dressing and clothing storage areas, and offices should be laid out to minimize dangers and distractions to gymnasts.

A gymnastic instructor or coach should take the following steps in planning:

1. Select desired activities and estimate number of participants by age groups.
2. Make tentative selection of needed apparatus (see Chapter 3).
3. Make tentative layout of apparatus, using checklist below and architectural drawings of gymnasium.
4. List required building alterations and special equipment for safety of gymnasts (see checklist and Chapters 4 to 6).
5. Estimate personnel needs for supervision, spotting, and maintenance (see Chapters 3 to 5).
6. Calculate cost and budgetary feasibility of all of the above.

7. Draft final program: activities and staffing schedule, apparatus and equipment lists, and gymnasium layout.

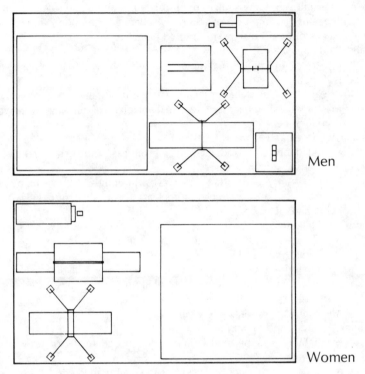

Men

Women

Sample layouts for an area of 50'×90'

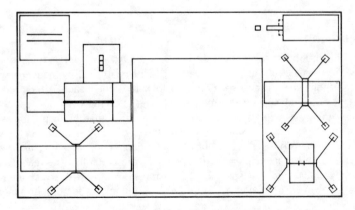

Layout for the 1977 American Cup in Madison Square Garden. Area is 57½'×104'

Checklist of Building Features for Gymnastics

Areas Including Runways and Walkways

In there adequate space for gymnasts, supervisors, visitors, and spectators? Especially are there straight unobstructed runways and safe dismount areas? Are active gymnastic areas properly separated from non-gymnastic areas by means of barriers, signs, or colored paint?

Walls, Partitions, and Obstructions

If there is any chance that a gymnast will collide with a wall or obstruction, is it properly padded?

Are all partitions stable or clearly labeled if unstable?

Are ropes and cables visible and kept clear of runways, walkways, and dismount areas?

Doors, Windows, and Mirrors

Are all doorways, windows, and mirrors safely located in relation to runways and dismount areas?

If there is any chance that a gymnast will collide with a window, door, or mirror, is it safely constructed (for instance, with shatterproof glass), properly hung, and clearly marked?

Floors and Platforms

Are floor specifications available for use in selection and installation of apparatus, mats, and safety devices?

Are platforms (raised areas) located where they will not overlap runways and dismount areas? Are edges of platforms safely constructed and clearly marked?

Are floorplate cut-outs safely constructed?

Lighting, Heating, and Plumbing Fixtures

Are lighting, heating, and plumbing fixtures adequate for gymnasts' health and safety needs?

Are utility control panels accessible and clearly marked?

Are fixtures safely installed and shielded when contact by gymnasts is possible?

Supervision

Supervision is one of the critical elements in safety, and reference to appropriate supervision is made throughout the various chapters. Ordinarily there are two types of supervision, general and specific, and to know when each is required is very important. General supervision means that one is giving overall direction to the activities going on, while specific supervision requires that the instructor be with a participant directly supervising the activity the participant is doing. In Chapter 11 on Legal Responsibility there is further definition of the meaning and scope of supervision, and that chapter should be read very carefully. The reader can also pull out various ideas on specific supervision from almost every chapter in this manual; however, following are some general guidelines for proper supervision.

1. Being present at all times for every activity of the program.
2. Developing a plan of supervision by rotating, observing, and communicating.
3. Inspecting equipment, watching for potential problems, anticipating errors.

4. Making sure that every assistant supervisor has proper credentials and competency.
5. Keeping people alert and motivated and under a controlled type of discipline.
6. Observing individuals from a physiological and psychological point of view, knowing when fatigue is setting in, or when activities are being performed irregularly or with too much force or speed.
7. Communicating with precise, understandable language so all know what is being said.
8. Seeing that participants know the rules and also follow them.
9. Overseeing from a nearby or moving position and not from a sitting or distant spot.
10. Making sure that after-school or after-class activities, if they occur, are carefully supervised or, if they are not to occur, that the gymnasium is locked or patrolled. Lawsuits are often traced to improper supervision. It behooves all teachers to be sure that they are well protected by functioning according to the best practices of supervision.

Supervisor-Gymnast Ratios

A ratio of instructors or coaches to gymnastic learners is difficult to specify because of the many variables, such as age, available equipment, skill level, sex of students, teaching methods, and teacher experience.

In some situations, in order to teach a fair volume of students and keep hazards at a minimum, teachers use compulsory exercises or skills of graduated difficulty and only allow students to advance from level to level on the basis of scores. Such a program could be made reasonably safe assuming that physical development and mental awareness coincide with score achievements. The circuit method of teaching under a controlled lesson plan or a compulsory exercise program has proven efficient in some circumstances.

Some events are by nature one-at-a-time activities, such as rings, vault, uneven parallel bars. A teacher may choose to plan a lesson in which several pieces of different apparatus are used in an effort to increase efficiency. It is worthwhile to assume that a single teacher will reach a "hazard level" if too many pieces of equipment are used at one time.

Gymnastic Programs: Four Types

Following is a general discussion of four types of gymnastic program. Each has its value and can be effective if administered correctly. Each also has its weaknesses, which must be considered when planning and implementing the program.

Mass Gymnastic Instruction Defined as more than eight gymnastic students in a class, this type of program is run in such a manner that the coach-instructor must control the class as a whole and has very little time, if any, to work with students on an individual basis. This situation is typical of public school or organization gymnastic programs. Under these circumstances spotting must be at a minimum, and a wide range of physical abilities may be present in the same class. A teacher-coach may have a considerable number of such classes per week and may need to rely more on written records than on memory to keep track of each participant's ability and progress (see Chapters 8 and 9). Program design and progressions must minimize those skills which have high risk factors and need individual attention.

Semi-Private Instruction Defined as two to eight gymnasts per class, where the instructor works with each student in turn on an individual basis, this situation is representative of private gym schools, clubs, and camps. Under these circumstances spotting is readily available if necessary, and the range of abilities is fairly consistent. The teacher-coach usually is well acquainted with each student's ability, as well as his/her strengths and weaknesses. Program and selection of skills can and should be designed to fully utilize the instructor-coach's individual attention.

Private Instruction Here one instructor works with one student over an extended period of weeks or months. Under this situation, which is ideal, the instructor knows in detail each student's abilities, strengths, and weaknesses.

The Team, A Special Situation Whether the team operates as a work-out, a class, or a class work-out, it requires special mention. Many clubs require scores or skill achievement to qualify for a team, thus assuring a certain homogeneity of skill level. In many cases, the basic skills have already been learned, and the practice revolves around the combining of skills into routines under strict supervision of the coach. When new skills are to be learned, they are under the control and guidance of the coach, who determines whether the individual is ready for such skills.

College or university teams sometimes permit beginners and advanced performers to practice side by side. The beginners should have demonstrated unusual natural talents in pre-testing. Such participants are under careful supervision by the coach and should follow a prescribed progression in their learning of all the necessary basic skills. This type of program can be justified for adults who are capable of self-motivation and making reasonable judgments about safety that young children may be too inexperienced to make.

1. Students should be required to successfully and safely execute specific skills or routines before proceeding to movements of recognized higher difficulty.
2. Students lacking in physical preparedness and strength should be identified and given practice limitations.
3. Assistant coaches or teaching aides should be required to demonstrate proficiency.
4. Coaches and their staffs should qualify for USGSA Certification as covered in Chapter 12.

Whatever the type of program, its overall goals must be established—and periodically reviewed—at the director's level. The program should have consistency. Periodic review of a program is necessary for continued upgrading, success, and safety.

3

Selection, Assembly, Installation, Care, and Maintenance of Gymnastic Apparatus

Selection—Look and Look Before You Leap

Choosing the right gymnastic apparatus for a particular program is an important and complex responsibility, although even the best equipment is no substitute for competent teaching and supervision. Following are suggestions, based on experience, for selecting apparatus.

Before you start shopping around, take a good look at your gymnastic program and define your needs. What activities are planned or likely to develop? Who will be using the apparatus? How old are these persons? How fit are they? Is this apparatus for beginners or for conditioned athletes in competition?

Once you know what your current and future needs are, you can begin researching all the available apparatus to meet those needs. Set your standards high. Select quality equipment from a reputable manufacturer. Your gymnasium is no place for marginal equipment.

Safety First. Any activity involving motion or height demands attention to safety precautions. The proper apparatus should be overbuilt—designed to provide generous safety margins.

Performance. Whatever the gymnastic activity, the apparatus should provide relative stability and, at the same time, optimum resilience when needed. Furthermore, it should provide an appropriate "feel" that enhances a gymnast's performance.

Durability. Your gymnasium apparatus is not a passing thing. It must be designed and built for years of rugged use. And it should be flexible enough in design to allow updating for future improvements and rule changes.

Adjustability. Check the apparatus for ease of adjustment. You may be changing height and/or width frequently, and you will want to make changes easily and quickly. Most importantly, the adjustment system should provide a dependable locking function to secure the apparatus once changes have been made.

Portability. See that your floor apparatus is a good traveler. You may have to move it from one gym to another as well as into and out of storage. It is best if one or two persons can easily take it down and transport it.

Convertability. Wherever possible, you should attach your apparatus to the floor. But be sure each piece of apparatus is easily convertible to a free-standing unit that does not require outside support.

International Specifications. Most competitive gymnastics in the U.S.A. are subject to rules and specifications established by various associations. Before you buy any apparatus for competition, see that it meets or exceeds these specifications.

FIG Specifications for Balance Beam

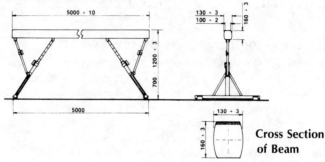

Cross Section
of Beam

FIG Specifications for Parallel Bars

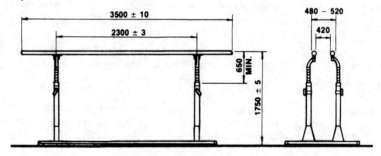

FIG Specifications for Horizontal Bar

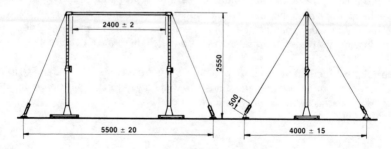

FIG Specifications for Vaulting and Pommel Horse

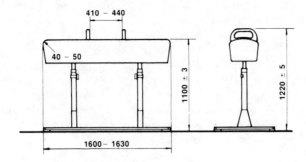

FIG Specifications for Uneven Parallel Bars

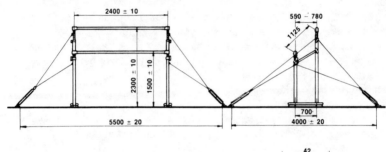

Cross Section of Bar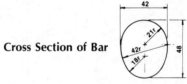

FIG Specifications for Rings

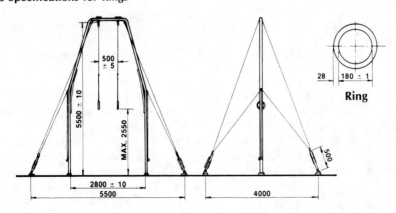

Ring

Assembly and Installation—Labors of Love and Patience

In order to become knowledgeable about apparatus, the instructor or coach should read all information obtainable from the manufacturer. If possible, the instructor or coach should direct or help with the assembling and should file the instructions for future reference.

Apparatus should be assembled exactly according to the manufacturer's instructions. If any questions arise, the manufacturer or his representative should be contacted.

If apparatus requires permanent installation or floor plates, experienced personnel should handle the job. Floor plates and wall and ceiling attachments are critical to safety and performance and demand expert workmanship.

Equipment Care—A Stitch in Time

Following are seven rules for daily care—or preventive maintenance—of gymnastic apparatus:

Take a good long look at your new apparatus and commit yourself to maintaining that like-new condition to assure safety and economy.

Learn and follow the manufacturer's recommendations for care of apparatus.

Check adjustment mechanisms and joints regularly. Keep them clean and lubricated.

Keep the finish clean.

After cleaning wooden parts, wipe dry with a cloth.

Find a good storage home for any apparatus made with wood. If your gym or storeroom allows wide variation in humidity, it could cause delamination or warping.

Never store wood products in or near the furnace area.

Safety Maintenance—Constant Vigilance

A comprehensive *Safety Inspection Checklist* is included below to assist in semi-monthly inspections, or whenever apparatus is to be subjected to heavy use during a meet or exhibition. In addition, the instructor/coach, as well as every gymnast using the apparatus, should develop an eye and a feel for a "just right" condition.

Use the apparatus only for its intended purpose.

Always follow the manufacturer's recommendations for use and maintenance of apparatus.

Carefully plan and prepare before moving the equipment. Even the slightest accident in moving the apparatus from one spot to another could damage critical parts and cause injury.

Encourage a special vigilance by all concerned when gymnasts are working out. It should be everybody's responsibility to stay alert for loose fittings and improperly adjusted equipment.

Keep an eye on friction points—wherever two or more parts rub together. Pay special attention to climbing rope fittings, cables, pullies, straps, bearings, protection pads, and swiveling joints.

Stay alert for loose fittings, set screws, bolts, and lock nuts. Equipment may feature joints designed with set screws or bolts to allow compensation for excess wear. Where necessary, apply a commercial "lock-tight" solution to keep set screws, nuts, and bolts from working loose.

Employ a light touch with tightening devices and turnbuckles. Forcing or over-tightening these adjustment devices can quickly cause stripping of the threads and eventual failure. Cover exposed bolt ends.

Keep in mind that any threaded joint realizes its fullest strength when all of the threads are being utilized. Letting a turnbuckle out to the point at which only a few threads are holding invites stripping and collapse.

Establish a routine inspection schedule for all critical parts of the equipment. Use a *Safety Inspection Checklist* similar to the one printed here to assure regular maintenance and attention to critical details.

If you are using more than one piece of the same type of equipment, assign each unit a number on the sheet and paint or stamp that number on the apparatus itself. When you make your inspection, enter a mark for OK or an R for repair or replacement. Be sure to make clear and detailed notations about the condition of each element of the apparatus.

Remove any doubtful equipment from service immediately and make sure it is not used until the condition is corrected.

Safety Inspection Checklist

UNIT NUMBER   COMMENTS

Item   #1 #2 #3

1. *Location of Apparatus* (should be suitable dis-
   tance from wall, sharp corners on chairs,
   benches, etc.). Keep in mind that a person
   landing off balance may take a few steps and
   then fall.
   A. Rings_____
   B. Horizontal Bar _____
   C. Pommel Horse _____
   D. Parallel Bar (men and women)_____
   E. Tumbling Mats_____
   F. Free Exercise Area_____
   G. Vaulting Horse_____
   H. Climbing Ropes_____
   I. Mats Placed to Eliminate Crevices ____
   J. Buck or Vaulting Box_____
   K. Beam _____
   L. Miscellaneous _____

2. *Safety Equipment*
   A. Hand Belts
      1. Condition of main body of belt_____
      2. Condition of all stitching—buckle to
         belt, sliding pad to webbing_____

    3. Condition of webbing where ring to rope
       contacts webbing⎯⎯⎯⎯⎯⎯⎯⎯⎯⎯⎯⎯⎯

    4. Rope snaps and rope attachment to snap ⎯⎯⎯⎯⎯

  B. Overhead spotting suspension

    1. Girder clamp—bolts tight ⎯⎯⎯⎯⎯⎯⎯⎯⎯⎯⎯

    2. If a traveling suspension, metal-to-metal
       wear of hooks, turnbuckle, and cable⎯⎯⎯⎯⎯⎯

    3. Condition of pulleys—grease pulley-
       wheel axles ⎯⎯⎯⎯⎯⎯⎯⎯⎯⎯⎯⎯⎯⎯⎯⎯⎯

    4. Condition of rope ⎯⎯⎯⎯⎯⎯⎯⎯⎯⎯⎯⎯⎯⎯⎯

    5. Belt (see 2-A) ⎯⎯⎯⎯⎯⎯⎯⎯⎯⎯⎯⎯⎯⎯⎯⎯

3. *Horizontal Bar*

  A. Examine bar for evidence of a "set" down-
     ward bend of the bar. Test with the bar UN-
     MOUNTED by using a straight edge or
     tightly stretched chalk line. If permanent set
     is more than ½", bar should be replaced.
     Under no circumstances should you reverse
     the bar.⎯⎯⎯⎯⎯⎯⎯⎯⎯⎯⎯⎯⎯⎯⎯⎯⎯⎯⎯

  B. If bar is adjustable, examine efficiency of
     pin for height adjustment and knob for tight-
     ening height adjustment pin ⎯⎯⎯⎯⎯⎯⎯⎯⎯

  C. Fastening of horizontal bar to vertical sup-
     ports (examine pins or bolts) ⎯⎯⎯⎯⎯⎯⎯⎯⎯

  D. Fastening of cables to uprights⎯⎯⎯⎯⎯⎯⎯⎯⎯

  E. Condition of cables (and chain), look for
     cable damage ⎯⎯⎯⎯⎯⎯⎯⎯⎯⎯⎯⎯⎯⎯⎯⎯

  F. Fastening of cables to end hardware (turn-
     buckles)⎯⎯⎯⎯⎯⎯⎯⎯⎯⎯⎯⎯⎯⎯⎯⎯⎯⎯⎯

  G. Condition of hooks and turnbuckles⎯⎯⎯⎯⎯⎯

  H. Floor plates (watch during workout for any
     signs of loosening) ⎯⎯⎯⎯⎯⎯⎯⎯⎯⎯⎯⎯⎯⎯

4. *Rings*

  A. Test clamps which are fastened to girders
     (tight, no play)⎯⎯⎯⎯⎯⎯⎯⎯⎯⎯⎯⎯⎯⎯⎯⎯

  B. Examine all hardware between girder and rings⎯⎯⎯⎯⎯

  C. Examine cable for wear and ropes for fray-
     ing (replace ropes that show aging—old
     fibers are easily torn) ⎯⎯⎯⎯⎯⎯⎯⎯⎯⎯⎯⎯⎯

  D. Condition of webbing and buckles and
     hooks on rings ⎯⎯⎯⎯⎯⎯⎯⎯⎯⎯⎯⎯⎯⎯⎯⎯

  E. If adjustable rings:

    1. Examine wall fastening bolts (no play)⎯⎯⎯⎯⎯⎯

    2. Examine fastening for chain ⎯⎯⎯⎯⎯⎯⎯⎯⎯⎯

    3. Examine chain ⎯⎯⎯⎯⎯⎯⎯⎯⎯⎯⎯⎯⎯⎯⎯⎯

    4. Condition of chain to rope fastener and rope itself_____

    5. Pulleys—oil axles, examine all parts for wear and all fastenings to wall or ceiling _____

5. *Climbing Rope*

    A. Clamp to girder or beam; all fastenings and entire unit solid (no play)_____

    B. Examine carefully all hardware between clamp to girder and the rope_____

    C. Examine rope carefully at hardware contact points_____

    D. Examine length of rope for fraying and old age_____

6. *Parallel Bars (men and women)*

    A. Note condition of bars. If bars are wooden and cracking occurs, rub in boiled linseed oil, wipe off excess, allow to dry 3 days, then lightly sand and chalk bar. If bars are fibreglass covered by wooden veneer, check for cracks or peeling in the veneer and contact the manufacturer about repair and replacement. _____

    B. Note especially metal fastenings to wooden bar (no play)_____

    C. Examine height and width adjustment_____

    D. All nuts, bolts, and screws (tight and no play) _____

    E. Rollers free of lint, easily raised and lowered (if built into base); lightly grease caster swivel for ease of movement_____

    F. Examine pads under base to prevent slipping and to protect floor_____

7. *Mats*

Check all edges, handles, tufting, sewing and note wear_____

8. *Pommel Horse*

    A. Check pommel surfaces _____

    B. Check fasteners which hold pommels tight_____

    C. Condition of body of horse _____

    D. Fasteners of body to base _____

    E. Height adjustment mechanism_____

    F. Rubber base pads _____

9. *Buck*

    A. Condition of body_____

    B. Fasteners of body to base _____

Item   #1   #2   #3

   C. Height adjustment mechanism _____

   D. Rubber base pads _____

10. *Vaulting Board*

   A. Condition of wood—any splits or breaks _____

   B. Take-off surface rough enough to prevent slipping; if surface is covered with carpeting, make sure it is securely fastened to board. _____

   C. Examine all screws and bolts _____

11. *Vaulting Box*

   A. Top surface firm and intact _____

   B. Examine joints for solidity, wood surface for splits or breaks _____

12. *Beam*

   A. Check beam surfaces _____

   B. Height adjustment mechanism _____

   C. Rubber base pads _____

4

Selection, Installation, Care, and Maintenance of Gymnasium Mats

Mats are a key element in gymnastic safety since they cushion both the gymnasium floor and other parts of the building, as well as parts of the apparatus, in order to protect the gymnast against injury from contact with hard surfaces.

Selection

Selection of mats should be made with five factors in mind: (1) the gymnastic activities planned, (2) the ages and fitness of the participants, (3) the nature of the gymnasium and the apparatus, (4) the continuing effectiveness of the mats themselves, given proper installation, care, and maintenance and (5) requirements of rule-making bodies. Good judgment also must be used. For instance, a mat suitable for floor exercises is inadequate for landing from a bar; a mat approved for competition may be unsafe for beginners; and a safe mat may become unsafe through abuse or neglect.

The FIG, USGF, NCAA, NHSF, and AIAW recommendations for mats in relation to specific gymnastic activities are summarized below. The NCAA mat specifications for Championship Meets should be consulted when a gymnasium is to be used for intercollegiate competition. In addition, the gymnastic instructor or coach must consider the conditions in a particular gymnasium, including provisions for care, storage, and maintenance.

A Basic Mat is used beside and under apparatus, or for floor exercises. A Base Filler (or Cut-Out) Mat fits around the base of the parallel bars and the pommel horse. The cushioning material of a Basic or Base Filler Mat should be firm. A Landing Mat is used in the landing areas for rings, horizontal bars, parallel bars, beam and vaulting horses, so it contains both firm and soft cushioning material. Special Mats are used to provide additional safety and reassurance for young children and beginners, or for experienced gymnasts learning new skills, so these usually contain only soft spongelike cushioning material.

Mats should be selected both in terms of their functional suitability and also in terms of durability and hygiene. If both covering and cushioning materials are resistant to water, rotting and bacterial growth will be inhibited. Most mats are enclosed in fabric envelopes, although some Basic Mats simply have painted exterior surfaces. Mat covers should give good traction, should be in colors that afford visual contrasts, and should fit tightly. Stitches should be made with durable thread and in places with minimal impact by gymnasts. Mat covers should be easy to clean, to repair, and to remove when replacement of cushioning materials is necessary. Some mats have adhesive end surfaces so that they can be fastened together.

Mat specifications at the Olympic Games (FIG) and at the NCAA Championships differ somewhat. In the case of the FIG the assumption is that gymnasts at this top level of competition are proficient and not in the learning stages; therefore the emphasis is on a firm base mat, with restrictions on additional mats. This base mat usually covers the entire competitive area. The cost of such a layout is enormous. World and Olympic Games specs (FIG) do not allow for landing mats under the rings or for the parallel bars. A landing mat is now permissible for vaulting, uneven parallel bars, and beam dismounts.

The NCAA, on the other hand, recommends that mats should provide a maximum amount of protection for the gymnast. U.S. rule-making bodies generally require more matting than do international bodies. The recommendations regarding sizes and thicknesses of padded areas around and under gymnastic apparatus are made primarily to assure that a proper working height from the floor to the working position of each piece of apparatus is provided. Landing mats are permitted over base mats for rings, parallel bars, vaulting, and horizontal bar. The 42' x 42' floor exercise pad is made of base mat. For latest recommendations and rules on mats, refer to the FIG Code and the NCAA Gymnastic Rules.

Installation

Supports and building obstructions should be covered by mats—properly cut-out when necessary. Lumps and gaps should be avoided. Basic Mats should not overlap. Special Mats should be placed over Basic and Landing Mats when appropriate.

Care

Gymnastic mats should be used only for gymnastic activities. Walking on them with improper footwear should be discouraged. Preventive maintenance will prolong the lives of mats and make them safer. Chalk and other dirt should be removed before it builds up, and adhesive end surfaces should not be overlooked. When mats are cleaned with soap or disinfectant, they should be wiped with clear water and dried.

Maintenance

Mats should be cleaned and repaired at regular intervals. Svitching should get particular attention. Torn covers should be mended or replaced, and "flattened out" cushioning material should be replaced. Cushioning materials should be selected not only in terms of their functional suitability but also in terms of durability. A record should be kept of original purchase dates and dates of repairs.

Safety Tips about Gymnasium Mats

1. Mats and protective equipment are not the complete answer to eliminating or reducing injuries. It is more important that falls be prevented rather than to assume that the fall will occur.
2. Careless progression or escalating learning at the expense of control and ability cannot be safeguarded by additional mats.

3. Landing on the head or landing in an out-of-control position can result in injuries regardless of extra mats.
4. Some good common sense and logic needs to be exercised in determining the size and number of mats needed for a particular activity.
5. Absolute mat requirements cannot be set for every situation, but the difference between resiliency and shock-absorbancy should be understood.
6. In a gymnasium, mats should never be idle. There is always a place for additional mats.
7. Mats are not fail-safe. Nothing can substitute for proper instruction, spotting, and good common sense in the teaching of gymnastics.

NCAA Mat Specifications for National Championship Meets

ARTICLE 1

It is recommended that all mats provided for use in gymnastic competition be constructed of high quality materials that provide a maximum amount of protection for the gymnast. The following recommendations regarding sizes and thicknesses of padded areas around and under gymnastic apparatus are made primarily to assure that a proper working height from the floor to the working position of each piece of apparatus is provided. All landing mats must provide a firm top surface.

ARTICLE 2

Mats provided for the side horse and parallel bars shall be so constructed so as to provide a level top surface without noticeable raised portions in the mat where it lies over and around the apparatus base members.

ARTICLE 3

Definitions and specifications of mats

a. Basic Mats

A Basic Mat is used around and under gymnastic apparatus. It is sometimes used in conjunction with a Landing Mat or a Base Filler Mat. It is constructed of a firm cushioning material and is designed to provide good protection for the gymnast. Two styles are in general use.
1. A fabric envelope exterior with a cushioning material or
2. A cushioning material with a painted exterior.
Basic Mats shall be 1¼'' ± ¼'' in thickness. The length and width of Basic Mats shall be ± 6'' of the designated dimensions in the following specifications.

b. Landing Mats

A Landing Mat is used in the landing areas under or near the rings, horizontal bar and the long horse. A Landing Mat is usually used over a basic mat to further cushion the gymnast's landing when dismounting from or vaulting over the apparatus. It is constructed of a combination of cushioning materials that result in a mat that provides maximum personal protection to the gymnast but, on landing, feels softer than a Basic Mat. It is constructed of a cushioning material interior and a fabric envelope exterior.

A Landing Mat is 8' ± 6'' wide x 12' ± 6'' long. Its thickness is 3¾'' ± ½''. The interior cushioning material of the mat consists of 1¼'' ± ¼'' of firm material and 2½'' ± ¼'' of a soft material.

c. Base Filler Mats

A Base Filler Mat is used to fill in the areas around the bases of parallel bars and pommel horse and its thickness is designed to equal the height of the base of the apparatus. When in place, these mats provide a raised landing surface around the apparatus that is flush with the top surface of the base of the apparatus. Basic Mats are placed on top of Base Filler Mats and when these Basic Mats are in place, no bulges are apparent where the Basic Mat covers the metal base of the apparatus.

Base Filler Mats are constructed of firm cushioning material. They are usually used under Basic Mats but sometimes they are attached to or are an integral part of the overlying Basic Mats.

ARTICLE 4 — FLOOR EXERCISE

The floor exercise area shall be padded. This padded area shall be 42' ± 6'' wide x 42' ± 6'' long and shall have a maximum thickness of 1½''. It is suggested that this padded area shall have a minimum thickness of 1''.

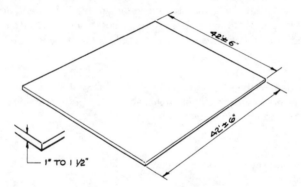

ARTICLE 5 — POMMEL HORSE

The pommel horse shall stand centered in a padded area made up of Basic Mats and Basic Filler Mats. This padded area shall be 12' ± 6'' wide x 12' ± 6'' long and shall have a thickness of 3¼'' ± ½''.

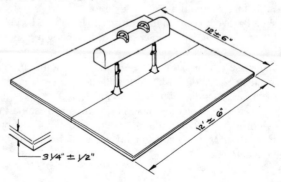

ARTICLE 6 — RINGS

The rings shall stand centered over a padded area made up of a Basic Mat 8' ± 6'' wide x 18' ± 6'' long centered under a Landing Mat 8' ± 6'' wide x 12' ± 6'' long. A second basic mat may be placed over the landing mat for additional safety. The total thickness of the combined mats shall be 6'' ± ¾''.

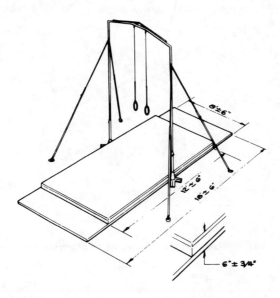

ARTICLE 7 — LONG HORSE

The long horse landing area shall be padded with a Basic Mat 8' ± 6'' wide x 18' ± 6'' long under two Landing Mats 8' ± 6'' wide x 12' ± 6'' long. The total thickness of the combined mats shall be 9'' ± ¾''.

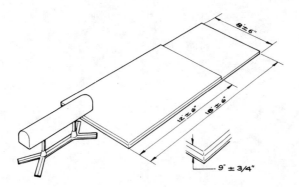

ARTICLE 8 — PARALLEL BARS

The parallel bars shall stand centered in a padded area made up of Basic Mats and Base Filler Mats. This padded area shall be 14' ± 6'' wide x 16' ± 6'' long and shall have a thickness of 3¼'' ± ½''. Provisions shall be made to allow a section of the padded area at both ends of the parallel bar to be removed completely to allow a Vaulting Board to be placed on the floor at either end for mounting purposes. Also, two 12' x 6' landing mats are to be available for the sides. Total mat thickness allowed for parallel bars is 7¼'' ± ¾''.

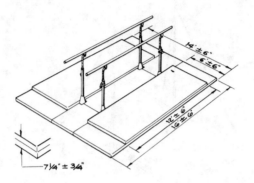

ARTICLE 9 — HORIZONTAL BAR

The horizontal bar shall stand centered over a Basic Mat 8' ± 6'' wide x 36' ± 6'' long. The landing area on both sides of the bar may be further padded with two Landing Mats 8' ± 6'' wide x 12' ± 6'' long on each side. The total thickness of the combined Basic and Landing Mats shall be 9'' ± ¾''.

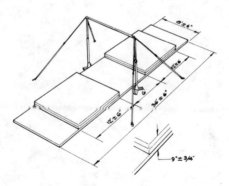

Suggested USGF Women's Mat Specifications

HORSE VAULTING

The horse vaulting landing area shall be padded with a basic mat a minimum of 6' wide x a minimum of 18' long under a landing mat a minimum of 6' wide x a maximum of 12' long. The total thickness of the combined mats shall be 5'' (± ¾'').

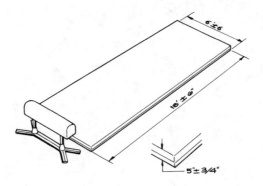

BALANCE BEAM

The balance beam shall stand centered in basic mats covering a minimum area of 12' wide. Entire area between bases must be covered. Any combination of basic mats to cover this overall area can be used. One 6' x 12' basic mat shall be used at each end. A landing mat shall be provided in the landing area with a minimum dimension of 6' wide x 12' long. The total thickness of the combined basic and landing mat shall be 5'' (± ¾'').

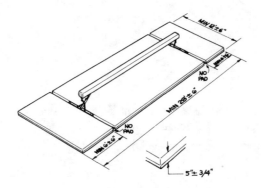

UNEVEN BARS

The uneven bars shall stand centered over a basic mat a minimum of 6' wide x a minimum of 30' long. A landing mat shall be provided. Landing mat to be a minimum of 6' wide x a minimum of 12' long. The total thickness of the combined basic and landing mats shall be 5'' (± ¾'').

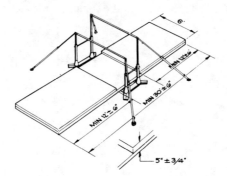

FLOOR EXERCISE

The floor exercise area shall be padded. This padded area shall be 42' wide (± 6'') x 42' long (± 6''). The top shall be joined into one continuous surface. The mat shall be a minimum of 1'' thick and maximum of 1½''.

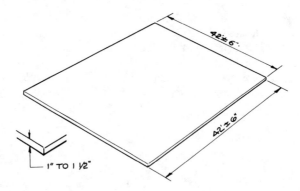

All basic mats shall be 1¼'' (± ¼'') thick.

All landing mats shall be 3¾'' (± ½'') thick with a minimum size 6' x 12'. If these mats fold, it shall be at the ¼ and ¾ length marks.

NOTE: No overlapping of basic mats will be allowed.

Recommended Competition Mat Specifications for Men

	FIG & USGF	NCAA	NHSF*
Floor Exercise:	54 mm thick	12000 mm × 12000 mm minimum 1″ thick	39′ 4½″ × 39′ 4½″ minimum ½″ thick
Pommel Horse:	12′ × 12′ base platform	12′ × 12′ platform filler minimum 3″ thick	bases should be covered to provide smooth landing area
Rings:	6″ maximum thickness for still rings base platform—8′ × 8′	base platform—8′ × 18′ one 8′ × 12′ landing mat 4″ thick (one additional 4″ landing mat allowable, maximum thickness—10″ total)	adequate mat cover maximum 10″ thick
Vaulting:	6″ maximum	8′ × 18′ base mat, 1¼″ thick (two 8′ × 12′ landing mats) 10″ maximum limit for all mats	adequate mat cover—maximum 10″ thick
Parallel Bars:	14′ × 16′ base platform mat	14′ × 16′ base platform mat minimum 3″ thick, extra 4″ landing mat 6′ × 12′ allowable up to 8″ maximum thickness	bases should be covered to provide smooth landing area
Horizontal Bar:	8′ × 36′ base platform mat— maximum 6″ thick	two 8′ × 18′ base mats, plus two 8′ × 12′ landing mats on each side (additional landing mats 8′ × 12′ × 4″ allowable on each side). Maximum thickness should not exceed 10″	adequate mat cover 10″ maximum thickness

Recommended Competition Mat Specifications for Women

	FIG & USGF	AIAW	NHSF*
Balance Beam:	two 6′ × 15 ½′ base mats fitted under beam, two 6′ × 12′ end base mats, one 4″ thick landing mat at either end	same as FIG, USGF	1¼″ base mat one 4″ landing mat
Vaulting:	6′ × 18′ base mat one 6′ × 12′ × 4″ thick landing mat	same as FIG, USGF	1¼″ base mat 4″ landing mat
Uneven Parallel Bars:	two 7½′ × 12′ base mats, one 4″ thick landing mat— 6′ × 12′ minimum	same as FIG, USGF	1¼″ base mat 4″ landing mat
Free Exercise:	54 mm thick 12000 mm × 12000 mm	minimum 1″ thick 12000 mm × 12000 mm	³/₁₆″ minimum thick

*NHSF—National High School Federation plans to issue more precise specifications in the near future.

5

Spotting Methods
and
Safety Equipment

Spotting is the technique of observing and assisting a gymnastic participant in order to facilitate the learning of skills and to minimize the risks of mistakes. Spotting is an essential part of assuring a safe progression of gymnastic skills at all levels of ability.

In planning a gymnastic program the instructor or coach must consider the availability of qualified spotters in relation to (1) the activities planned; (2) the number, age, and experience of participants; and (3) the apparatus and safety equipment available. The need for special mats—such as crash mats and foam pits—and for special aparatus—such as low balance beams, rings, and bars—is dictated as much by the nature of available spotters as by the nature of participants. And the need for special safety equipment—such as hand or overhead belts— assumes not only gymnasts who need them but also spotters who can use them.

The procedures for selection, installation, care, and maintenance of special safety equipment are the same as those for apparatus. The gymnastic coach or instructor has the same responsibility for adequate, properly functioning safety equipment as for everything else in the gymnastic program.

In a class situation, physical education teachers should teach the techniques of spotting and should require adequate practice in spotting skills. Students can then spot for each other in the beginning stages. This is both good training for the students and efficient, since one teacher cannot safely spot for the entire class. When using student spotters for beginning skills, the teacher must remember their limitations of age, size, strength and ability. Responsibility for safety is always the teacher's, not the student spotter's. For more advanced skills spotting should be done by persons with additional training and experience in the various methods of spotting.

The observant spotter should anticipate possible problems and be ready to cope with them. Doing this requires knowledge of the various skills being performed. The observant spotter will watch the gymnast's head, which is a key to control of motion; the hands, for signs of a loose or slipping grip; and the facial expression for an indication that the performer is losing control or lacks confidence. In short, the spotter must have the necessary strength, experience, and, above all, involvement.

An effective spotter should hold the performer's complete trust and confidence. This trust is gained only after repeated experiences of spotting and assisting gymnasts through a wide range of skills. An efficient spotter must be totally immersed in the performer's actions, anticipating any variations which may cause a mistake or fall. An "on the alert" attitude must be maintained constantly. The performer must feel confident that the spotter has control at all times. With this confidence, the performer can concentrate on the skill.

The four common methods of spotting are Hand; Hand Belt; Overhead Traveling Belt; and Overhead Mounted Belt.

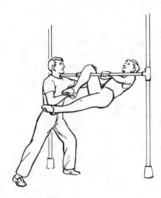

Hand Spotting

Hand spotting is spotting with the hands alone. This method is widely used, particularly at beginning levels, because it does not require the gymnast to get into a belt or the spotter to get the ropes ready. Many gymnasts and coaches prefer hand spotting because it frees the spotter to lift, manipulate, turn, or catch a performer without being involved in holding a rope. Also, it enables a spotter to effectively block a gymnast, thus sending him/her up into the air for the proper set action prior to executing a twist or somersault, while the spotter remains ready to assist the gymnast to land safely. It takes an alert, strong, and experienced spotter to spot effectively with the hands, but those who are qualified prefer hand spotting to any other method. Hand spotting is not limited to tumbling and balancing skills. It can be used for the parallel bars, high bar, rings, vaulting, balance beam, and uneven bars.

In hand spotting, the spotter shold be close to the performer and even be in contact if possible. The goal in protective spotting is to control the action. While a gymnast is first learning a move, contact should be made even if it proves to be unnecessary. Sometimes it is difficult to make contact if the gymnast has lost control and is flailing with arms and legs. For some skills two spotters are desirable. The spotters must know where to stand to be most effective. This will vary according to the apparatus and the skill being performed. In general, the spotter should position himself between the performer and the place on the floor where the performer is most likely to land. Most spotters stand too far away. A person can fall quickly, and unless the spotter can move in to catch him/her the spotting safeguard is useless. however, the spotter should not stand so close as to hamper the performer or to expose the spotter himself to injury or collision. Another reason for standing close is leverage. If it is necessary for a spotter to catch a gymnast who is falling, it will be more difficult to stop the fall at arm's length than from closer to the performer.

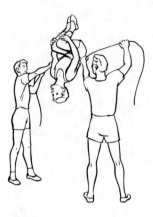

Hand Belt Spotting

Hand belt spotting involves attaching a belt around the performer's waist with ropes extending from each side for use of the spotters. This method is useful for such skills as back handsprings, back saltos, front handsprings, front saltos, round-off flip flops, and the like. Students can be taught to spot with the hand belt and entrusted up to intermediate levels of skill. For such spotting to be effective, the ropes must be grasped close to the gymnast for maximum leverage. For running passes, the ropes should be held loosely during the run so as not to interfere with the performer but grasped tightly as the skill is performed. If a running pass is used into a round-off and a twisting belt is not available, the ropes will have to be brought across the body in such a way as to unwind when the round-off is performed.

Overhead Traveling Belt Spotting

This method requires the installation of two parallel cables overhead approximately twenty feet apart and fifty feet long, on which running pulleys can be attached so a tumbler may perform down the stretch with the pulleys and ropes riding along with him. As the spotter becomes efficient the gymnast may start away from the anchor point, allowing for longer run into the tumbling area. The spotter "lets out" several feet of rope and then rapidly retrieves it as the tumbler runs into the tumbling area. This method takes practice since the inexperienced spotter's hands may slip or miss the rope as it is pulled into action. The ropes must be kept fairly taut to make the pulleys travel along the cables. The spotter should stay even with or slightly ahead of the performer in order to facilitate the movement of the pulleys. The Pond Twisting Belt is especially effective with this type of rigging, although a web belt may be used with a crossing of ropes for moves such as round-offs, Arabian dives,

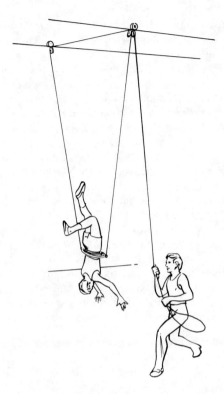

and the like. Timing is important while spotting with the overhead traveling belt so that the lift is made at the proper moment. Also the force of the lift varies—being greater for a back somersault than for a back handspring and even stronger for double backs and/or twisting movements. It is imperative that the ropes leading from the overhead pulleys to the sides of the belt remain taut enough to keep the performer's arm from becoming entangled. For many activities the overhead traveling belt system is an effective method of spotting.

Overhead Mounted Belt Spotting

This method requires pulleys attached to an overhead beam through which passes the rope for the belt. Most gymnastic rooms have belts over the parallel bars, rings, trampoline, balance beam, uneven bars, and high bar. For all apparatus except the horizontal bar the belt is fixed directly overhead, whereas for the high bar the point of suspension is generally a few feet in front of the bar (this also may be true for the uneven bars).

Some general principles to follow in using an overhead mounted belt are:

1. Always look to make sure the ropes are hanging properly and not tangled. With experience this checking should become an automatic reflex.
2. Do not pull too tightly on the ropes while the gymnast is getting into position on the high bar, parallel bars, rings, or uneven bars. This can impede the

gymnast's swing to a handstand, cast to a layaway, or the like, thus interfering with the pending skill. Start with the ropes in an untight position and then, as the performer swings into the move, tighten the ropes for effective spotting. This method differs in tumbling, where a taut rope is essential throughout the activity.

3. Stay with the gymnast as he completes an activity, by keeping pressure on the ropes, thus helping him/her to a controlled landing. Above all, do not relax the rope and then give a last pull, driving the belt uncomfortably into the gymnast's stomach.

4. Always check on the proper number of times for the rope to encircle the high bar if the gymnast plans a giant swing or two before dismounting. A coach needs only one experience of having too many wraps around the bar prior to a dismount to implant deeply in his mind the need to check the correct number of circles of the ropes. Also check closely on the proper direction of the ropes for reverse flyaways, regular flyaways, vaults, hechts, and the like.

5. When spotting a gymnast on the rings, allow the rope to slide through the hands as moves like giant swings, giant bails to dismounts, and the like are tried. This procedure takes practice since it is imperative that the spotter's hands are constantly in contact with the ropes and ready for an effective spot. Also be sure to know where and when at the bottom of the swing you should pull the ropes to assist the performer upward into the balance of the giant swing, double flyaway, or the like.

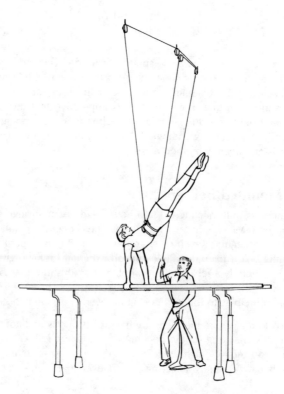

6. Remember that an effective spotter is one who constantly has the ropes in a "ready position" and yet not in a tight carrying position throughout a move. This rule should be qualified somewhat in that during the early learning stages the coach may want to carry an athlete through a move. As skill progresses the gymnast should develop an increasing feeling of doing a move on his own, thus the slight "letting-up" of the ropes by the spotter—but remember always to keep the ropes in a ready-to-save position.
7. Note that overhead belt can be used effectively to pull a performer off the side of the parallel bars for a single or double back dismount. The technique is to pull one rope more strongly than the other toward the dismounting side.

Concluding Guidelines for Effective Spotting

1. Be constantly alert, anticipating incorrect movements which will necessitate rescuing of the performer through either hand or belt spotting.
2. Watch the gymnast carefully, anticipating an early or late release which could cause trouble and necessitate an active step in spotting or an efficient pull of the overhead belt.
3. Follow the gymnast all the way through the skill including the landing.
4. Do not hesitate to overspot a gymnast, especially during the early learning stages, rather than to underspot.
5. Whenever a reasonable doubt enters your mind regarding the safety of a gymnast, take appropriate spotting action at once.
6. Consider wearing golf gloves while spotting with an overhead belt. The soft pliable leather gives good adhesion and prevents burning of the hands due to friction.

Spotting is an essential part of assuring the proper progression of gymnastic skills. Many gymnasts and even some teachers and coaches are reluctant to get involved in learning the science of spotting due to apprehension, but it is only by trying that a person can learn. A person can learn to spot. Progression needs to be incorporated so that the spotter becomes familiar with a proper sequence of techniques, methods, and procedures. Learning can be aided by the instruction and supervision of a qualified and reputable person with experience and knowledge of spotting activities.

Supplementary Gymnastic Safety Equipment

1. Spotting Belt
2. Twisting Belt
3. Overhead Suspension (Permanent)
4. Overhead Suspension (Traveling)
5. Suspension (Horizontal Bar)
6. Landing Mat (4")
7. Crash Mat (6" through 12")
8. Training Pad (Balance Beam and Uneven Bar)
9. Wall Pad Paneling
10. Spotting Block (Various Sizes and Weights)

11. Low Balance Beam
12. Low Rings
13. Low Parallel Bars
14. Low Horizontal Bar
15. Landing Pits

6

Personal Equipment:
Clothes and Accessories,
Chalk, Hand Guards

The word *gymnastics* comes from the classical Greek *gymnazein,* meaning to train naked. The word's origin emphasizes the point that every item of a gymnast's bodily attire should be considered with respect to safety. Does the garment or accessory make the gymnast more or less safe? Special personal items such as chalk, hand guards, and tape come to mind first in connection with gymnastic safety; but clothing, footwear, glasses, jewelry, and hair or nail styles are equally important.

Clothes and Accessories

Clothing. In practice, the gymnast should wear a garment that is fairly light in weight and that allows complete freedom of movement without being too loose-fitting. For women, the leotard is ideal; it allows maximum range of motion, is very light in weight, and fits the body tightly. To protect the arms and legs from abrasions and to keep warm, commercially sold "warm-up suits" are recommended. These suits fit tightly around the wrists, ankles, and waist, insuring that the clothing will not fall into the gymnast's line of sight when she is upside down or become caught between the apparatus and the gymnast's hands or feet. Normal sweat clothes can serve the same purpose as warm-up suits, but care must be taken to avoid excessively baggy clothing that may blind the gymnast or become entangled with the apparatus. A bra is generally considered a needed protection for women.

Men usually wear a leotard-like step-in jersey for competition, but prefer more informal attire for daily practice. An athletic supporter should be worn at all times along with a pair of not too baggy shorts and a T-shirt of some kind. Pants with belt loops are not recommended, and belts with buckles should never be worn. In addition to the possibility of getting caught on something, a belt buckle may damage the apparatus. Form or warm-up pants can be held up with suspenders, and care should be taken to insure that the suspenders are strong enough to hold during strenuous activity.

Footwear. Footwear for gymnasts comes in many different styles and is partly a matter of personal taste, provided functional safety is considered. Some prefer to work barefoot, some prefer socks alone, and others prefer a gymnastic slipper. Because of the greater possibility of stubbing a toe or of spreading germs, working without some type of foot covering is not recommended. Gymnastic slippers or booties are ideal for balance beam, floor exercise, and vaulting. Slippers are lightweight and are usually made of nylon, canvas, or leather with varying types of soles. A heavy-duty leather or canvas type is preferred for vaulting, while the very lightweight cotton footie type is often preferred for the balance beam. Other kinds of athletic footwear such as sneakers are generally too cumbersome for safe gymnastic work.

Jewelry and Glasses. All jewelry should be removed before participation in gymnastic activity. Hanging earrings could catch on the apparatus, and a necklace could fly in a gymnast's face, temporarily blinding or distracting her. Rings, watches, and bracelets will not only prevent an optimum grip, but also may cut into the skin or into the apparatus. When glasses must be worn, care should be taken to be sure they are securely fastened around the head. Many gymnasts find contact lenses ideal for gymnastics work.

Grooming. Gymnasts must show more concern for their personal grooming than most athletes. In competition the gymnast is judged partly on appearance during an event, and long hair that is not tied back can distract from an otherwise quality performance. More importantly, however, is the danger involved when hair momentarily blocks a gymnast's line of sight or inhibits a hand placement. It is crucial, therefore, that hair be cut short or tied back securely when a gymnast is performing even the most basic skills. Finger- and toenails should be kept short enough to avoid interference with gripping or footing, as well as self-inflicted scratches.

Chalk and Handguards

Magnesium Carbonate. Commonly referred to as "chalk" or "mag," magnesium carbonate is used on a gymnast's hands to absorb perspiration. Most athletes are concerned with foot traction, and many different types of shoes have been designed to prevent athletes from slipping on various kinds of surfaces. The gymnast, however, spends a large portion of his time on his hands, and must keep them relatively dry if he hopes to stay in contact with the apparatus. Attempting to perform on the horizontal bar with sweaty hands would be as foolish as scaling a mountain cliff in the rain with smooth leather-soled boots. Sweaty hands not only endanger the gymnast at fault, but also make the apparatus slippery for those who follow. Magnesium carbonate helps prevent blisters by reducing the friction between the hands and the apparatus to a slight degree, but its primary purpose is just the opposite: to keep the hands dry and insure a good grip.

Chalk can be purchased in small blocks or as a powder. Caution should be taken when using either form of chalk to keep the powder on the hands or in a container designed for holding it. Too much chalk in the air can make a gymnastic area very unpleasant, and too much chalk on the hands may cause excess powder to get in a gymnast's or his spotter's eyes.

Rock rosin is an accepted material used by some performers on wood surfaces for better footing. When a beam is padded, rosin and chalk are not recommended.

Hand Guards. Also called palm guards or simply "grips," hand guards act as a protective device that separates sensitive skin from abrasive apparatus and allows a gymnast to work horizontal bar, still rings, pommel horse, parallel and uneven bars for extended periods of time. For the purpose of protecting the hands, most grips are placed over the palm by slipping the middle two fingers through holes and buckling the strap around the wrist. The rough surface of the grip should face away from the palm to provide better contact with the apparatus. In addition, the rough side will tend to hold chalk better than the smooth side. Hand guards come in many different shapes and styles and are made of several different types of material:

(1) WICK GRIPS

(2) LEATHER GRIPS

(3) SUEDE GRIPS

(4) SYNTHETIC GRIPS

(5) STRING GRIPS (one-piece hand grips used primarily by girls for uneven parallel bar work)

(6) RING GRIPS AND THE DOWEL: Recently, hand guards have been used to assist in holding the gymnast onto the apparatus in addition to simply providing protection for the hands. This purpose is accomplished on the still rings by a larger leather grip which is worn on the finger tips and includes a sewn-in dowel. The dowel creates a fold that fits around the ring.

The dowel is placed between the fingers and the ring and causes the fold which holds the hand to the ring. The dowel grip should be confined to advanced work, and its use should be evaluated by the instructor or coach. While this grip has advantages for very advanced ring work, the beginner may find that it causes difficulty in letting go of the rings upon dismounting, and must be cautioned to use the dowel grip only when working advanced stunts with close supervision.

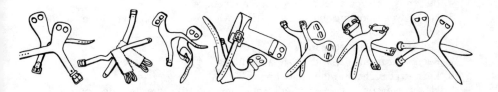

The same principle demonstrated with the ring grip is also used by many elite male gymnasts on the horizontal bar and by some on the parallel bars. A dowel is not usually used, but a normal leather grip is worn on the finger tips and a fold is worked into the leather as the grip is broken in. The purpose here is not so much to hold on easier, as to put more of the pressure on the grip and less on the hand, thereby allowing the gymnast to work the apparatus for a longer period of time.

Caution should be used in making a dowel grip or otherwise altering personal equipment.

All hand guards wear out in time. Depending on the quality of leather or other material used and the amount and type of use, a grip will last anywhere from a few weeks to several months. Grips should be inspected daily for any indication of weakness or tearing. Likely places for tearing are the center of the palm and the wrist strap. Leather grips will dry out with age and become somewhat brittle and slick. Any grip with a torn or slippery surface should be replaced immediately.

Additional Hand Protection. Gymnasts are often eager to practice in spite of very sore hands. For this reason tape is often used on the hands under hand guards. It is recommended that tape be run from the wrist to the fingers, rather than across the palm. This method of taping will lessen the chance of tape rolling up in bunches. Foam rubber may also be placed under hand guards to add another layer of protection between the hand and the apparatus. Two pairs of overlapping hand guards are even used on occasion by gymnasts with very tender hands. All of these methods of hand protection can be used safely if the user is cautious not to jeopardize his actual grip of the apparatus. The size of a person's hands will put a natural limit on the amount of protection that can be worn while still insuring a safe grip of the apparatus.

Fifteen Rules for Safe Outfitting

Gymnasts keep in contact with the apparatus primarily with their hands, their feet, and their eyes. Common sense leads to the conclusion that these three lines of contact must be kept free from interference in order to have safety in gymnastics. The following safety hints wil eliminate most of the risks caused by clothing and personal equipment.

1. Be sure your hair will not block your vision, no matter what your body position is. Remove gum, candy, etc., from your mouth.
2. Don't let the length of your finger- or toenails interfere with your grip or footing.
3. Never wear jewelry when performing.
4. Be sure your eyeglasses are securely fastened.
5. Never wear clothing that may interfere with your hands, your vision, or the spotter's vision.
6. Use appropriate footwear.
7. Keep your hands dry with chalk at all times.
8. Keep excess chalk in the chalk box.
9. Never use grips made of inferior materials, and be sure the grip you use is adequate for your purpose.
10. Check grips daily for weakened stitching, tears, and hard slippery surfaces.
11. Be sure grip buckles are fastened securely before performing.
12. Be sure the rough surface of the grip is in contact with the apparatus.
13. Never use dowel grips without expert supervision.
14. Never endanger your holding power with too much protective material on your hands.
15. Don't wear anything while you are performing that will interfere with normal gymnastic performance and the efficiency of spotting.

7

Visual Aids:
Wall Charts, Films, Still Pictures

Visual aids can enhance motor learning, if they are properly used. By helping the learner visualize an activity, visual aids can make learning more efficient. Visual aids also can increase the learner's motivation and confidence, thereby reducing fear. Teachers, coaches, and spotters can learn skills including spotting techniques with greater efficiency, motivation, and confidence by means of visual aids. Thus such materials contribute significantly to gymnastic safety.

Proper use of visual aids has two sides: first, selection of accurate materials; second, discussion by the learners. Accuracy is essential, since inaccurate details not only are distracting but may stick in the learner's mind at the expense of the points to be learned. Discussion is essential both to assure the learner's complete understanding of what he sees and also to reinforce verbally the visual stimulus. The instructor should use leading questions to be sure the discussion covers all essential points.

The three major kinds of visual aids used in gymnastic instruction are: films including movies, film strips, and videotapes; wall charts including lists of rules, apparatus and skill diagrams, progression charts, self-evaluation charts, and instructor's evaluation charts; and series of drawings or still photographs.

Films

Next to live demonstrations, moving pictures are the most effective means of teaching motor skills. Projection speed can be varied to emphasize a whole routine or a detail of technique. Moving pictures also have a high motivational and confidence-building effect.

Some commercial sources of films (8 or 16 mm., loop, or strip) are listed below. Amateur films of meets, clinics, and exhibitions can be borrowed from coaches or gymnastic enthusiasts. Videotaping can provide instant replays so that a gymnast gets immediate reinforcement of strengths and awareness of weaknesses.

The Athletic Institute
705 Merchandise Mart
Chicago, Ill. 60654

Abie Grossfeld
Gymnastic Coach
Southern Connecticut State College
New Haven, Conn. 06515

Donn Clegg
501 S. Highland Ave.
Champaign, Ill. 61820

Frank Endo
12200 S. Berendo Ave.
Los Angeles, Cal. 90044

Gymnastic Aides
Northbridge, Mass. 01534

Association Films, Inc.
561 Hill Grove Ave.
La Grange, Ill. 60525

Wall Charts

A most important wall chart is the Gymnastic Rules poster adopted by the USGSA and available from the Association or the gymnastic equipment companies.

The old-fashioned blackboard and mirror are still hard to beat for many purposes. With a blackboard (or sheets of newsprint) the instructor or coach can emphasize points by adding or erasing. By means of a mirror the gymnast can observe many aspects of his technique.

Diagrams of gymnastic skills, apparatus, and spotting techniques are available from such sources as those listed below—or can be locally developed by using available artistic and drafting talent.

Progression charts are invaluable visual reminders of proper learning sequences and warnings against by-passing essential basic skills. Charts containing self-evaluations and instructor's evaluations provide both motivation and challenge.

Gymnastic Aides—see above

WM Productions
PO Box 10573
Denver, Colorado 80210

AMF American Athletic Equipment Division
200 American Ave.
Jefferson, Iowa 50129

Nissen Corporation
930 27th Ave., S.W.
Cedar Rapids, Iowa 52406

Still Pictures

Drawings, diagrams, and photographs of gymnastic activities in sequence are the most readily available visual aids—and the least expensive to obtain and use. They can be found in magazines, catalogues, and books or prepared locally. With imagination still pictures can be presented in appealing ways: shelved or racked in reading rooms or corners, collected in albums, or mounted on posters. Some of the many sources are listed below.

International Gymnast
Sundby Sports Publications
PO Box 110
Santa Monica, Cal. 90406

Gymnastics Illustrated
Don Tonry
Hoctor Productions
Waldwick, N.J. 07463

Conditioning for Gymnastics
Bob Spackman
Hillcrest House
Carbondale, Ill.

Gymnastic World
Sundby Sports Publications
410 Broadway
Santa Monica, Cal. 90405

Sportswomen-Books
Market Place
PO Box 1293
Los Altos, Cal. 94022

Code of Points
USGF
PO Box 12713
Tucson, Arizona 85711

Gymnastics for Men, for Women
A. Bruce Frederick
Wm. C. Brown Co.
Dubuque, Iowa

Feminine Gymnastics
Burgess Publishing Co.
Minneapolis, Minn. 55435

Note

Gymnasts' attention must be called to the USGSA Gymnastic Rules poster on p. 40. Recent legal cases have increased the supervisor's responsibility to make sure participants *understand* risks involved in an activity (see p. 109).

GYMNASTICS RULES

1. *Caution:* Any activity involving motion, rotation, or height may cause serious accidental injury.
2. Do not use apparatus without qualified supervision.
3. Wear proper attire and use chalk when necessary to prevent slipping.
4. Before mounting apparatus, make sure it is properly adjusted and secured, and that sufficient mats, appropriate to the exercise, are in position. Consult your instructor.
5. Use proper conditioning and warm-up exercises before attempting new and/or vigorous moves.
6. Attempt new skills in proper progression. Consult your instructor.
7. When attempting a new or difficult skill, a qualified spotter should be used. When in doubt, always use a spotter—check with your instructor first.
8. Dismounts from apparatus require proper landing techniques. Do not land on head or back as serious injury may result. Consult your instructor.
9. Any skill involving the inversion of the body could be dangerous and cause serious neck or head injury.
10. NO "HORSE PLAY" AT ANY TIME WHILE ON OR AROUND GYMNASTICS EQUIPMENT.

8

Physical Preparedness
and Warm-up Exercises

The instructor or coach bears much of the moral and legal responsibility for the physical preparedness of participants in a gymnastic program. This responsibility is shared with the administration of a school, college, university, or other organization, and with designated medical personnel. It also is shared with the participant or his/her parent or guardian. But the instructor or coach has the most important share of responsibility for physical preparedness—including the responsibility to make sure others do their share. The following steps should be taken with respect to all participants' physical preparedness in order to assure the safest possible program:

1. *Require periodic physical examinations and maintain accessible medical records.* The kind of physical examination required for gymnastic participation usually is prescribed by one or more of the following: state law; regulations of school district, college, university, or organization; rules of interscholastic or intercollegiate athletic association. The examination must be made by a licensed physician. The instructor or coach must know what kind of physical examination is required for his program and at what intervals—and, in the rare case when he considers the examination inadequate, must report the inadequacy to proper authority. He/she must keep a Medical Information Form on every participant where it is readily available for consultation in case of emergency (see Chapter 10, Medical Responsibility in the Gymnasium).

2. *Discuss physical examinations with participants (or parents/guardians of minors).* The instructor or coach should discuss the medical examination report with every would-be participant (or parent/guardian) in the event of disqualification or doubt about participation in gymnastics because of a physical condition, so there will be full understanding by all concerned. If the participant wears glasses, the need for safe lenses and frames and for securing-devices should be discussed, and the possibility of contact lenses might be broached. If the participant is overweight, he/she might be advised to discuss diet with a physician. Need should be stressed for full information about a participant's chronic ailments in the event of an emergency (see Chapter 10). The handicap of a missing bodily part or organ—such as an eye, a kidney, a testicle, or fingers or toes—should be explained so that waivers are not signed casually.

3. *Require consent, waiver, and release forms and keep them on file.* A consent form should be on file for every gymnastic participant, signed by parent or legal guardian if the participant is a minor, or by the participant. The form should contain a waiver of claims against the sponsor and staff of the gymnastic program for any aggravation of a pre-existing condition, or for any injury

resulting from that condition. The form also should release the program's sponsor and staff from responsibility for any injury occurring during the program. Consent, waiver, and release forms are frequently prescribed by educational institutions and athletic associations or clubs. It should be recognized that such forms are primarily for public relations purposes and that a participant consents *only* to the "normal" risks of the sport, and that in signing a form does not waive the right to sue for negligence. The supervising instructor/coach should consult a lawyer in case of doubt about the forms.

4. *Establish a testing program to record participants' physical preparedness and skill level at all times.* The best measure of a gymnastic participant's physical preparedness to learn a skill is his/her ability to perform a more basic skill. In other words, a gymnastic testing program should be related to progressive teaching of skills (see Chapter 9). The charts that follow present first skill tests for both boys and girls, designed to determine readiness for Level One, the beginning level, of any gymnastic activity. These tests give norms for age levels from 6 to 22, but the top norms can be extended to persons in good physical condition up to age 40—and beyond if used with discretion. For participants with no gymnastic experience, three sessions of preparation are recommended for the Level One Readiness Tests. Tests for higher skill levels should be based on the activity progressions in Chapter 9. A class chart or file can be used to record the participants' progression from level to level. In a large class or group, participants' skill levels can be indicated by color dots, arm bands, or other visual codes on their apparel.

5. *Appropriate warm-up exercises should be taught with skills and required before every activity.* Gymnastic participants should be reminded constantly of the importance to their safety of proper warm-up. General physical preparedness and mastery of skills do not remove the risk in starting an activity "cold." Every instructor and coach should prescribe a set of warm-up exercises for each activity, and make sure these are done. In addition, each participant's strengths and weaknesses should be assessed periodically, and special exercises should be prescribed to correct weaknesses. In the next section is a set of basic warm-up exercises that has been effective in a successful gymnastic program. The value of dance training for gymnasts is advocated by many experts, so a section on that topic ends this chapter. It presents a series of dance exercises for both general conditioning and warm-up.

Note: The above steps—including required physical examinations and consent, waiver, release forms—are not a guarantee against damage suits for alleged negligence, but following them would help convince a judge or jury of the instructor or coach's intent to conduct a responsible and safety-conscious gymnastic program (see Chapter 11, Legal Responsibility in the Gymnasium).

Gymnastic Readiness Test (Males)

No.	Description of Skill	Ages: 6–9	10–14	15–18	19–22
1	Pull-ups—from straight hang to chin over bar	3	6	8	10
2	Push-ups—prone position, body rigid on rise	8	15	20	30
3	Standing Broad Jump—toe to heel	4'	5'	6'-7"	7'-2"
4	V Balance—body and legs form 90 degrees	3 sec	5 sec	7 sec	10 sec
5	Handstand against the Wall	3 sec	5 sec	10 sec	25 sec
6	Forward Roll and Straddle Leg Roll-up	Bent Knees	Slightly Bent	Straight Knees	Straight Knees
7	Horizontal Bar Undershoot—bar 5'	3'	4'	4'-10"	5'
8	Touch Head to Knees, Grab Ankles—hold position	1 sec	2 sec	3 sec	3 sec
9	Rope Climb, Hands and Feet	10'	15'	20'	20'
10	Rope Climb, Hands Only	4'	8'	15'	20'
11	Rope Skipping (one hop per rotation)	5 sec	10 sec	20 sec	30 sec
12	Parallel Bar Push-ups	½	2	5	7
13	L Hang on Rings and Hold	1 sec	2 sec	3 sec	4 sec
14	Touch Hands to Floor—knees straight	Finger Tips	Palms on Floor	Palms on Floor	2 sec Hold Floor

15	2-Arm Cartwheel —for form	Bent Legs	Slightly Bent	Straight Legs	Straight Legs
16	L-Support on Horse—straight legs	½ sec Hold	2 sec	3 sec	4 sec
17	Backroll Recovery	Tuck	Straight Legs	¾ Handstd	Thru Handstd
18	Headstands	3 sec	5 sec	Clap Hands Recovery	Same
19	Bridge	Hold 3 sec	Support 25 lbs	Support 100 lbs	Support 125 lbs
20	Sit-ups, Hands Back of Neck	30	50	60	70
21	Front Vault (use appropriate height)	Low Horse Height	¾ Horse Height	Normal	High Front Vault
22	Squat Balance	2 sec	5 sec	10 sec	10 sec
23	40″ Wand Double Hop	Hop One Foot At Time	Double Hop Over	Hop Over & Back	Same
24	Forward Rolls	Tuck Roll	Off One Leg	Bounce Dive	Same
25	Front Pullover on Horizontal Bar	Chest High	Bar at Reach Height	Jump Height	Same

Some Possible Rules:

Each skill worth 4 points when completed and card punched by teacher.

Perfect score listed as 100: 25 × 4.

Recommend 3 periods devoted to practicing skills.

On test day, second attempts permitted.

Recommend that record cards be filed in gym office for 5 years.

Ages:	6–9	10–14	15–18	19–22
Persons recording successful attainment of the following scores can be considered to be of very good physical preparedness:	80–100	80–100	84–100	88–100
Satisfactory physical preparedness for:	60–79	64–79	68–83	68–87
Fair physical preparedness for:	40–59	48–63	56–67	56–67
Poor physical preparedness:	below 40	below 48	below 56	below 56

Note: Some of the norms were taken from studies by the President's Council on Physical fitness and the Canadian Association for Health, P.E. and Recreation.

Gymnastic Readiness Test (Females)

No.	Description of Skills	Ages:	6–9	10–12	13–15	16–22
1	Flexed Arm Hang (chin above bar) and hold		10 sec	20 sec	20 sec	25 sec
2	Push-ups		10	20	25	30
3	Standing Broad Jump		3'-7"	4'-4"	4'-10"	5'-2"
4	Sit-ups		10	25	30	40
5	V Balance		3 sec	5 sec	7 sec	10 sec
6	Handstand against the Wall		3 sec	5 sec	10 sec	25 sec
7	Touch Head to Knees and Hold		1 sec	2 sec	3 sec	3 sec
8	Rope Skipping (1 hop per circle)		5 sec	10 sec	20 sec	30 sec

#	Skill				
9	2-Arm Cartwheel	Slightly Bent Knees	Straight Legs	Same	Same
10	1-Arm Cartwheel	Slight Knee Bend	Straight Legs	Same	Same
11	Headstand	Against Wall	Free	Clap Hands Recovery	Same
12	Bridge (hold 2 sec)				Same
13	Forward Front Scale	2 sec	3 sec	4 sec	5 sec
14	Front Vault (Swedish box, horse)	Low	Medium	Normal Height	Same
15	Forward Roll	Bent Knees	Straight Legs	Dive Roll	Same
16	Straddle Roll Split	High Split	6" Split	2" Split	Same
17	Front Hip Pull-over	From Kick Over	From a Stand Position	Same	Same
18	L-Support Position	1 sec	2 sec	3 sec	3 sec
19	Beam Walk, Hop	Walk Length	Hop Length	Slide Steps	Slide Steps
20	German Hang Return	On Low Bar	On Reach Bar	On High Bar	On High Bar
21	Momentary Handstand —split legs return	Hold 1 sec	2 sec	2 sec	2 sec
22	Arch-jump Control Landing	Controlled Landing	Same	No Steps	No Steps

23	L-Hang on the Bars and hold		1 sec	2 sec	3 sec	3 sec
24	Back Roll to Single-knee Balance		Bent knee roll	Pike roll	Same	Same
25	On Beam Jump to Mount to Stand (SIT-LIE-SIT-STAND)		once	once	once	once

Some Possible Rules:

Minimum requirements are listed and performers need not exceed this number to get credit for that skill.

Each skill completed is worth 4 points—25 × 4 equals 100, perfect score.

For new students never exposed to the activity, have a three-period preparatory session prior to testing.

On the test day second attempts should be permitted.

Test cards can be punched in appropriate boxes for later tallying.

Suggest that test cards be maintained in the instructor's files for five years.

	Ages:	6–9	10–14	15–18	19–22
Persons recording successful attainment of the following can be considered to be of very good physical preparedness:		80–100	80–100	84–100	88–100
Satisfactory physical preparedness for:		60–79	60–79	68–83	68–87
Fair physical preparedness for:		40–59	40–59	48–67	52–67
Poor physical preparedness:		under 40	under 40	under 48	under 52

Basic Warm-up Exercises

Proper warm-up exercises add to both the safety and the success of every gymnastic activity. Many warm-up systems have been advanced; the following is simply one based on years of instruction and competition. Every instructor or coach should prescribe a warm-up routine for each gymnast, based on periodic reviews of his/her strengths and weaknesses. There is no sharp line between general conditioning and warm-up exercises. The former are taken when a need is recognized; the latter are taken routinely even if a gymnast feels "in great shape." The value to the gymnast of studying dance, whether classical or modern, should be noted here (see next section).

(1) Start all workouts by stretching, limbering, and flexing the entire body. Get in the habit of pointing the toes. This not only develops a good habit, but also stretches the feet and legs. Be careful that correct alignment is maintained, and that the foot does not sickle.

(2) Begin standing with arms above head, toes straight ahead (parallel); keeping knees tight, bend forward and reach toes; slowly come up with arms over head, and lean back, stretching the upper back slowly.

(3) Standing with feet apart and turned out, bend from the waist sidewise, right and left; then execute a circle, starting by bending to the right, reaching the floor, and coming up left to an upright position. Repeat several times.

(4) Feet together, slowly do several releves, rising onto ball of the feet; repeat with turned-out feet.

(5) Standing, bring one leg up to a bent position, clasp with both hands and pull knee tight; hold for several counts. Repeat with other leg.

(6) Swing arms up and back, taking time to thoroughly flex shoulder area.

(7) Include easy running in place. Remember to point toes while running.

(8) Sitting on floor, legs in front together, stretch forward, slowly reaching toes (pointed). Do this several times; then repeat with flexed feet. Knees are kept straight and tight.

(9) In sitting position, legs apart as far as possible, stretch as far forward as you can, with chest leading. Do not arch back. Repeat with flexed toes, several times.

(10) Bend knees in a "tuck" position, tight; clasp each ankle with hands and hold for 5 counts; release to a straight position, head to knees.

(11) Take same tuck position as in 10, and roll back and up to a standing position; repeat same tuck roll back and finish with a "walk out" standing.

(12) Lie flat on back, sit up to a V sit position, hold, lie back, and repeat.

(13) "Rocking chair": sitting with legs apart, reach forward to floor, then lie back and reach legs over head to reach the floor with both feet. Keep toes pointed, and feel stretch in spine.

(14) "Candle," or shoulder stand, legs together: roll down to sitting tuck then "bicycle" on candle position.

(15) Lying on tummy, arch backward slowly, keeping legs straight: then do the same with bent knees, trying to reach toes to head. Grasp ankles with hands, and gently try to straighten knees.

(16) On tummy push up to a knee scale, repeat with other leg, and include swan balance position.

(17) Lying flat on back, push up to a back bend slowly, taking time to stretch arms and knees, and gently rock forward and back. Repeat back bend from a standing position if capable.

(18) Heel stretches: sitting on floor, grasp instep of one leg and stretch it straight; repeat with other foot, then with both.

(19) Standing up, face wall or barre, kick leg behind, low at first, gradually increasing height. Repeat kicks to front and side.

(20) Place one leg on barre or a beam, keeping toes pointed; bend and try to reach chest on knee; hold, then repeat with toe flexed.

(21) Slowly execute a split on the floor, never trying to force; take time to stretch, and no bouncing. Repeat in all directions; be sure to do the "bad side" as well as the "good side."

(22) Handstand practice: remember arms shoulder width, never wider. Do several scissors handstands, then go to fully stretched position and stag handstands.

Dance Training for Gymnastic Safety

Proper dance training can be an invaluable aid in the safety and effectiveness of learning gymnastic skills and exercises. Gymnastics training focuses on activities requiring rather large movements involving intricate coordination combined with strength and agility. Dance works at the foundation level, creating a body awareness incorporating all the elements (agility, rhythm, flexibility, timing, etc.) which allow the gymnast to learn the more difficult movements necessary to complete the gymnastic skill.

Specific dance exercises teach the participant to move body parts in isolation, giving knowledge of muscle groupings and also increasing strength and flexibility. The dancer also concentrates on the body's central axis and on the lines or planes running vertically and horizontally through and around the body. Learning to move into and hold the various positions of ballet not only increases the participant's body awareness but also develops an effective sense of balance. Learning the basic elements of dance along with gymnastics also is an excellent way to improve concentration and discipline. Dance exercises require a patience which is too often lacking in gymnastics training.

Gymnastic conditioning and warm-up can borrow from the discipline, placement, stretching, and strengthening exercises of ballet. The dancer begins with placement and plies, centering the body around an axis, learning to extend and coordinate arm and leg movements to the front, side, and back, and concentrating on correctly supporting his weight during knee bends (plies). Thus he strengthens his muscles while at the same time learning to avoid stressful positions at the joints. Many gymnasts have experienced painful injuries to ankles, knees, and lower backs which might have been avoided if they knew and practiced correct placement.

Dance Exercises for General Conditioning or Warm-Up. Following is a sequence of dance exercises which can be used by gymnasts for conditioning or warm-up. The whole sequence can be completed in 20 or 30 minutes and, practiced regularly (at least 2 or 3 times per week), would be an aid for any gymnast interested in quality and overall physical awareness. These movements should be practiced with the aid of a bar for balance on the right and left side before attempting same movements in the center (without bar).

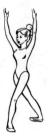

I. Plies
    A. Four grands plies in first, second, and third position
        1. rhythmically
        2. straight spine/flat stomach
        3. squared off hips and shoulders
        4. pelvis held straight, neither dropped forward nor tucked under
        5. heels down on first half of grand plie (demi plie) in first and third position, and heels down at all times in second position grand plie.
    B. Follow each set of four plies with a grand port de bras forward and backward.

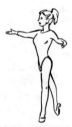

II. Tendue and degage (tendu: extending leg with pointed foot, toes touching floor; degage: extending leg through tendu with pointed foot leaving floor)
    A. To front, side, and back from first and third position
    B. Shifting weight and lowering heel from tendu to fourth position (tendu front or back) and second position (tendu side)
    C. Intermix with demi plies (heels remaining on floor)
    D. Follow with balances in releve in first and fifth position

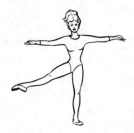

III. Developpe
    A. Passing through correct passe position extend leg to front, side, and back:
        1. maintain turnout, square off hips and shoulders at all times
        2. coordinate arm movements
            a. front for passe
            b. overhead for front developpe
            c. to the side for side developpe
            d. forward for back developpe
    B. May include holding leg in extended position and removing hand from bar for balance and/or include a releve
    C. Practice carrying leg from front extension to side and back and reverse (rond de jambe)

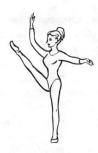 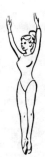

IV. Battements (Kicks)
    A. To front, side, and back from first and/or third position
        1. squared off hips and shoulders
        2. don't bend standing (support) leg
        3. coordinate arm position (see III. 2. above)
    B. Follow with grands plies and port de bras forward and backward while holding releve
V. Jumps
    A. Sixteen jumps from first position
        1. stretching feet to fully pointed position in the air
        2. using plie on take off and landing with heels touching floor at the bottom of plie
        3. maintain carriage of upper body and arms
    B. Sixteen changes alternating right foot forward, left foot forward in third position
    C. Eight jumps in second position

VI. Swings and basic body waves
    A.   Legs parallel
    B.   Using contracted stomach and supple spine

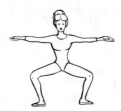

VII. Several grands plies in second position after the rest of workout is completed

To maximize the benefit of a ballet bar or any dance warm-up, it is not enough to simply go through the motions. The utmost concentration is necessary. One must concentrate on individual body parts and muscle groups as well as on the positions of the body as a whole. Certain lines must be found in the body, but their importance lies in their relationship to the whole position and the center of weight. Movement should not be static or machine-like; any movement can have life and feeling.

Concentration on good posture is the beginning of safe movement and simply means standing as tall as possible with a straight line running from the crown of the head down through the center of the body. To stand in this way, careful attention must be given to the shoulders and pelvic alignment. The shoulders should not be slumped or pulled back too far but should be centralized and relaxed so that the neck is long and without tension. One should also be careful not to carry one shoulder higher than the other, as is often the case with people who overtrain one side of their body. Good pelvic alignment means the upper body is supported directly on top of the legs for maximum height. When the pelvis is incorrectly tilted forward (a very common postural error) the weight of the upper body is carried in front of the legs, led by a weak stomach, causing a stressful and potentially dangerous condition in the lower back. Bad posture is a vicious circle, incorrect pelvic alignment being related to weak ankles, flat feet, and knock knees. Make a complete correction in any one of these areas and the other problems will also begin to disappear.

Another method of finding one's physical center and achieving good posture is to lift one's weight up through the legs (especially the inside muscles of the legs) and stomach while at the same time feeling the weight drop down from the head and shoulders but without sacrificing height. In this way concentration is brought into the solar plexis area of the body, the real physical center of the body's mass and weight. It is from this point that good balance is achieved.

A few minutes of each warm-up should be dedicated to feet, ankles, hands, and wrists. Slow stretched rotations in both directions repeated until there is some tiredness and slight aching in the wrists and ankles will strengthen and safeguard against injury. Another good exercise for feet and ankles is to practice flexing the toes independently of the foot and also to flex and point the whole foot. For the hands and wrists, a good practice is to alternately make a tight fist and then stretch the hands wide open, separating fingers as far as possible.

In all sorts of plies the relationship of the knee to the foot is especially important. Whenever the knee bends on a weight-supporting leg, the knee should extend over the foot, if possible over the small toe side of the foot. Otherwise the knee joint is in a vulnerable and weak position (knock knees) badly supported by the muscles of the leg.

Some people have another problem with the knee if they can hyperextend this joint. Hyperextension is beyond straight, tends to be a locked position and is very dangerous on landings. Gymnasts who have hyperextension should be aware of this condition and practice standing with the leg straight (this will feel slightly bent to them) rather than hyperextended.

After learning to stand in correct posture, the backward port de bras is an excellent exercise for gymnasts to improve their acrobatic work. With the arms extended overhead (one arm if using a bar) feel a straight line running through the body, then extend this line up and back, at the same time keeping the weight supported on the legs, lifting up through the legs, stomach, and lower back during the entire movement. The arched position must come from a feeling of length if it is to be correct and not pinch the lower back. With enough flexibility one can reach and look directly behind the body, making a 90 degree curve. Use stomach muscles and return to a straight line in the same rhythm used to go into the back bend. This exercise can be done with the legs parallel or turned out in first or second position and also with the legs turned out in third position.

These types of dance exercises practiced with some regularity, as part of a gymnast's general warm-up, will lead the gymnast into greater physical awareness, improve muscle control, and reduce the risk of injury during the rest of the gymnastic workout.

9

Progression in Teaching Skills

Experts in gymnastics around the world often say that learning of skills slowly and in a progressive manner is the single most important factor in success and safety. Over-spotting sometimes indicates that fundamentals are being bypassed and that a short-cut method of learning is in progress. Often such lack of skill progression points to unqualified instructors who have not systematically studied and listed a progression for each activity.

In order to help instructors in listing skills in progression from basic movements to the high intermediate level, the editors have asked experts in each activity to contribute their recommendations. Most accidents occur at the beginning and intermediate levels, where enthusiasm may outstrip ability and participants have not learned to "pace themselves" properly. But progressive learning should continue even at advanced or championship levels, and advanced progressions can be prepared from books in this manual's bibliography.

In spite of careful progression, no system can be completely foolproof. Since everyone learns at a different rate and since some students may be extremely talented while others are slow learners, the quick learners often unconsciously bypass some of the progression. Good judgment is also needed, for it takes an expert to decide whether to adhere to a rigid "ladder program" or to allow some exceptions.

Joseph Stalder of Switzerland, one of the greatest gymnastic technicians, said that one should not try to learn more than four new medium-difficult skills per year per event. His feeling stems from the fact that time should be less important than the perfection of new skills and the adequate development of the body.

An approximate guide to progressions for each activity is presented in this chapter. It is impossible to grade steps exactly because some gymnasts find a movement quite easy while others find it more difficult; but from the standpoint of safety, instructors should keep a check-off record for each participant. Bypassing one or two steps along the way is not as serious as a complete rejection of a systematic disciplined manner of learning. Skills bypassed should be returned to at later times.

Progression on one activity can be facilitated by appropriate steps in another activity. This type of concomitant learning has advantages for participants who become involved in an all around program. Progressive learning needs to be motivated by the instructor through compulsory exercise programs and various stimulating games and challenges. A qualified gymnastic instructor will insist on a progression program at the expense of a faster skill-learning progress. In the end he will be the victor. Instructors should temper the enthusiasm of each student with a realistic assessment of his or her resources of strength, skill, and courage. When teaching young people, it is advisable to vary the schedule for every training session so that much of it is a review of skills presented in a slightly different manner in order to keep up the enthusiasm of the participants.

Teaching Body Awareness

Beginning progressions should be devised to teach the gymnast body awareness. The following questions could be used as guidelines to test the gymnast's body awareness:

1. Does the gymnast have an awareness of general body position and of various parts of the body in relationship to the whole, based on internal cues (kinesthetic awareness)?
2. Does the gymnast realize the human body's structural limitations in relation to gymnastics—especially the dangers of excessive weight on the neck; lateral flexion of the knees or elbows; and undue strain on the spine, shoulders, ankles, and wrists?
3. Does the gymnast realize the need to *unlearn* instinctive reactions in some situations—for instance, closing eyes, thrusting hands out, letting body go limp?
4. Does the gymnast realize the importance of balance, including the fact that body positions which are unstable in a static position may become stable during movement?
5. Can the gymnast determine left and right when in an inverted position?
6. Can the gymnast determine where the limbs are in a number of varied body positions?
7. When approaching a particular skill, does the gymnast understand the appropriate tensions, extensions, or compressions involved?

Preparing a gymnast through progressions can eliminate or cut down on many potential hazards, but will not eliminate hazards completely. For instance, the gymnast can have tendencies, caused by fear, to stop short after initiating the beginning movements of a skill. To help avoid this problem, the instructor should be satisfied that the gymnast is committed and ready to accept that commitment and follow through. Should the gymnast follow through and not complete the skill properly, a spotter should be prepared to assist.

Teaching Landing and Recovery from Falls

Landing and recovery from falls are essential skills in all areas of gymnastics. They require a kinesthetic awareness different in degree from that required in other sports. The unique combination of speed and variety in gymnastic movements requires automatic reactions both in normal landings and also in abnormal falls.

Proper landing and recovery are fundamental movements that should be taught even before tumbling or vaulting. Maintaining body balance, proper use of arms and placement of feet, and correct use of leg muscles and joints, all need to be learned by most human beings. In addition, constant awareness of the danger of unexpected falls should be inculcated.

Two major areas of skill should be taught: landing on the feet from controlled jumps or dismounts; recovery landing from abnormal falls. Following are sets of drills for developing these two safety skill areas.

1. Warm-up drills can include
   a. rope skipping (on balls of feet),

b. jumping in place with tuck jump on fourth count,

c. jumping (after one or two steps) from take-off boards to mats, with emphasis on proper arm action in take-off and landing.

2. Landing technique explanation, demonstration, and practice (progressing from one-foot to two- and three-foot tables and then double tables).

a. Emphasize awareness of joints and muscles, especially the quadriceps (great extensor muscle of the front of thigh). Give special attention to knee bends *without hyperflexion of knee joints*. Caution against locking legs in landing from forward or backward jumps.

b. Give directed practice (preceded by explanation and demonstration) in jumping and landing, emphasizing proper use of arms and the slight knee bend which is adequate for soft landing.

c. Give directed practice in finding best positions of gymnast's body, arms, and feet for balance as well as appearance.

d. Give directed practice in placement of feet on the mat, emphasizing the use of an *almost* flatfooted landing for balance. Explain the disadvantage of landing only on balls of feet and trying to establish balance with improper use of ankle joints.

e. Give directed practice in landing from arch, squat, and straddle jumps, showing how straight controlled position is slightly modified; also in landing from backward jumps.

3. Recovery technique explanation, demonstration, and practice.

a. Emphasize the desirability of distributing the force created by the impact of landing over as many points of the body as possible—in most circumstances—rather than breaking a fall by absorbing the entire shock of impact with the hands, arms, feet, or knees. (Note extreme cases when a person may have to risk a limb to save his life.)

b. Give directed practice in falling forward to prone position on a mat, bending arms to absorb the shock. First fall with body and knees slightly bent, then with body and knees straight. Return to standing position by a hand walk.

c. Give directed practice in falling backward to cradle position on a mat, with hands behind and *fingers pointing forward toward the body* in order to allow elbow joints to hinge. Contact should be made first with hands, then with seat, and finally with back as roll ends at cradle position. Return roll to erect position is reverse of fall. Fall should be made in a forward body pike, first with knees slightly bent, then—when movement has been mastered—with legs straight for fall and return roll.

4. Handstand recovery movements. Before getting into the long process of developing a handstand, gymnasts should master the three common recovery movements used when the body moves beyond a vertical position.

a. Pivot recovery is made by reaching forward with the hand on the same side of the body as the lead kicking leg and turning the body in cartwheel style.

b. Arching over to a bridge position, absorbing falling shock with feet, is another form of handstand recovery. Hands should be held on mat until feet make initial contact.

c. A forward roll-out is made by bending the arms slowly to lower the body while tucking the head and body. At first spotters should hold the gymnast's legs and guide them through a controlled roll.

5. Progression of jumping drills for beginning gymnasts, designed to develop a safe distribution of force from the impact of an expected or unexpected landing. A soft matted area, protected against traffic and obstacles, should be provided for landing.

   a. Jump forward from a 6-inch height, landing on the feet and absorbing the impact by slightly flexing the knees.

   b. Jump forward from a 6-inch height, landing on the feet and immediately executing a forward shoulder roll while the arms form a protective "roll-cage" over the head (roll-cage position: chin tucked into chest).

   c. Jump backward from a 6-inch height, landing on the feet and then rolling backward to a cradle position while maintaining a roll cage with arms and head.

   d. Jump backward from a 6-inch height to a landing on the feet, then to a backward roll accepting body weight on the hands (placed behind body with fingers pointing toward body).

   e. Jump forward from a one-foot height, landing on the feet and immediately executing a forward shoulder roll without using hands or arms—except to maintain roll-cage position.

   f. Jump backward from a one-foot height, landing on the feet and rolling to the back cradle position while maintaining a roll cage.

   g. From standing position jump to a forward shoulder roll without using hands.

   h. Jump from about 3½ feet height, landing on the feet and absorbing impact through flexion of knees.

   i. Jump from about 3½ feet height, landing on the feet and immediately executing a forward shoulder roll while maintaining roll-cage position.

   j. From a squat position roll backward to a cradle position while maintaining a roll cage.

Tumbling and Floor Exercise: Areas of Concern

This activity should be approached both for its own values and also as the basis for many other phases of gymnastics. It sets the groundwork not only for the basic skills of recovery from falls but also for the highest-level skills found in one form or another in almost every event in the All Around program.

Of special concern is the *mat*. Is it smooth, with no gaps or holes? Is it clean, dry, and unslippery? Is there a "traffic police" system to keep the mat free of gymnasts from other activities, spectators, and too many participants claiming rights to the area (a special problem in tumbling and floor exercise because of the absence of apparatus)? Are enough extra mats, including special ones, used for beginning activities?

Adequate warm-up is a concern, because of the amount of body extension and contact pressure involved.

Experienced and responsible supervision is a special concern in tumbling and floor exercise. For one thing, an unusually high degree of hand spotting is required in this activity. For another, progression is a relatively subjective matter—depending on the judgment of the instructor/coach and the gymnast. The supervising instructor/coach should insist on adherence to a progression table, with no shortcutting of lead-up skills, recovery movements, and appreciation of risks. No student should be forced into an activity for which he is physically or gymnastically unprepared.

Safety Tips for Instructors and Coaches

1. Make sure the floor exercise or tumbling area is smooth, level, and free of obstructions. Check frequently for soft or flattened places and replace inadequate mats.
2. Provide extra spotting in the teaching of any skill that can involve pressure on the neck, especially among beginning gymnasts.
3. Make sure adequate spotting is provided in the teaching of running somersaults and other moving skills. This requires thorough communication between gymnast and spotter regarding the nature of the exercise and the exact starting point.
4. Insist on the development of upper body strength as well as leg power.
5. Don't forget spotting the landing on an aerial or somersaulting skill as well as the take-off.
6. Do not allow a gymnast to try to compensate for a physical weakness through improper technique (for instance, locking arms during a fall to compensate for lack of strength to support the body).
7. Avoid "pitching," throwing, or forcing students through skills that they are not physically or progressively ready to attempt.

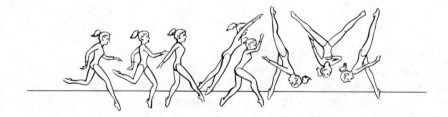

Tumbling and Floor Exercise Progression (Women)

Following is a suggested progression of some tumbling skills for girls or women, from basic skills to the medium difficult ones. Care should be taken on all take-offs and landings of sideward skills because of the weakness in the knee in the lateral motion.

Some spotting hints have been included. Where handspotting becomes less effective, do not hesitate to use hand belts for extra precaution. Although basic mat coverage is adequate for most of the skills, extra landing or crash mats will add security and confidence in the performer. Crash mats for somersaults in the early learning stages add safety to the program. Instructors must use good judgment in the use of mats and safety equipment.

Forward roll—A tuck roll starting on feet and ending on feet.
Spotting: Be sure roll is performed on the neck, not on the head.

Forward straddle roll — A roll finishing in a straddle standing position.
Spotting: Following the gymnast from behind, giving support on the hamstring area at the finish.

Forward pike roll—A straight leg roll requiring flexibility. It is not necessary to pike at the end.
Spotting: Spot from the side under the stomach as the roll is initiated to relieve pressure on the neck. The other hand may assist in putting the head under.

Headspring/neckspring kip extension—From the head or neck, a kipping action to an extended standing position.
Spotting: Spot from the side, one hand on the small of the back, the other on the upper arm. During the kip, the back-hand will support and help body extend, the shoulder-hand will work in opposition, forcing the gymnast to stay extended and also to prevent over-rotation.

Headspring kip squat—Same but ending in a standing squat.
Spotting: Same.

Handstand-forward roll—A roll from a handstand.
Spotting: Holding the ankles or legs, support the body as the head is turned under. This will help to eliminate a piking position during the roll.

Handstand-limber—From a handstand, arch to a backbend, then stand to feet.
Spotting: Spot from side—one hand on the small of the back, the other on the upper arm.

Walk over—From a split handstand, a forward one-leg support to the feet.
Spotting: Same.

Cartwheel—A handstand side ways in a straddle position, landing one foot at a time.
Spotting: Support on the hips until feet touch the floor.

One-arm cartwheel—Same but using either arm.
Spotting: Same.

Cartwheel/dive cartwheel—From a fast cartwheel there is a successive push from each knee as it touches the floor. The arms throw over the top of the body, reaching for the ground.

Spotting: As gymnast puts her second leg down on the 1st cartwheel, move hands to grasp her on the hips and lift and set her into the ground.

Roundoff—A cartwheel with a 2-leg landing facing the way you began.
Spotting: Hands on the hips, lift the gymnast through the turn to the feet.

Back extension roll—A back roll and quick arm extension to a handstand.
Spotter: As the roll is initiated, grasp the legs at the ankle or knee, lifting the gymnast to a handstand.

Back limber—From the feet, arching back to a backbend (bridge) and kicking both legs over to a standing position while passing through a handstand position.
Spotting: Lift the back as the gymnast's hands touch the floor, and shift the body over to a handstand by supporting the lower back and upper legs.

Front handspring—A skip step into a handstand, push from the hands extending over to the feet.
Spotting: Same as a front limber, but the hand on the back should be moved around the waist. Emphasis is on the push from the hands (shoulder block) and a strong straight leg kick—hand on the upper arm should be kept on to prevent over-rotation.

Front handspring walkout—Stepping out of a handspring.
Spotting: Same as a handspring—care should be taken to give a soft landing on the first leg, accomplished by a slight lift as the leg touches.

Tinsica—Beginning a cartwheel, the hands are staggered, finishing into a front walkover.
Spotting: Same as a handstand-limber.

Dive handspring or cartwheel—From the skip, the arms reach forward and up in a swinging motion as the front leg pushes the body up.
Spotting: The spot is accomplished after the arm swing. Same as a front handspring. Pressure must be taken off the arms by lifting the body slightly. Emphasis is on teaching the gymnast not to land on an extended arm!

Mounter—From a two-foot takeoff, the arms are over the head reaching down as the legs push the body up. The gymnast lands in a piked handstand and pushes immediately to a front walkover position.
Spotting: As the gymnast takes off, give support under the stomach to keep pressure off the arms.

Back handspring (flic flac) (flip flop)—From a stand, a back jump in an arch position to the hands, then a quick push from the hands to the feet.
Spotting: Caution must be used by beginning instructor *and* gymnast. Instructor must be strong enough to completely support the gymnast in his arms. With one arm around the gymnast, lift the gymnast as she reaches back. Set her into the floor in a handstand position, then shift an arm to the

stomach to prevent falling on the stomach if the feet do not get down quickly enough. As the gymnast develops an understanding and proficiency, the arm spot may move to a handspot. Constant care must be taken to keep the gymnast from a hard landing on the wrists and arms.

Back tinsica—A back walkover, landing on the hands one at a time in a cartwheel position.
>   *Spotting:* Same.

Back walkover—With the weight on one leg, the gymnast arches back to a handstand split and then to an arabesque (front scale), finally bringing the legs together.
>   *Spotting:* Teaching flexibility will help—lift the non-support leg up to at least 90° before she reaches back—insist on a 180° split during the handstand, support the lower back as the hands touch and shift to the stomach as gymnast passes through handstand.

Back walkover straddle through to straddle sit—Back walkover to handstand, straddle through the arms to a straddle sitting position.
>   *Spotting:* Spot as a back walkover, then shift to the back of the gymnast; standing over her, hold hips up as the legs drop to a straddle.

Roundoff flip flop—A front beginning into a cartwheel, double leg landing into an immediate backjump to handstand, push to feet.
>   *Spotting:* As the feet approach the ground on the roundoff, the arm moves into the back of the gymnast lifting her to the handstand. NOTE: If the roundoff is good and the flip flop is good, the gymnast can eventually learn the skill herself without a spot by decreasing the waiting time between the two skills.

Front somersault—From a 2-foot takeoff the arms are over the head, elbows slightly bent. The arms reach out and up, creating a thrust. The arms grasp the knees half-way through the skill. The landing is in a semisquat or stepout position.
>   *Spotting:* One arm under the stomach, the other on the shoulder. Stomach arm lifts, shoulder arm turns the gymnast.

Back somersault (flip)—Standing—A jump up and back to a tuck position, landing on the feet.
>   *Spotting:* One arm around the gymnast, one arm on the back of the leg. As she reaches, the spotter lifts her and turns her. As she lands, the arm shifts to the stomach to prevent over-rotation.

Back tuck somersault—A roll over the head in a tuck position.
>   *Spotting:* Lift the hips as the head makes contact with the floor.

Aerial cartwheel—From a one-leg takeoff a cartwheel without using the arms and landing on the leg that leaves the ground first.
>   *Spotting:* Same as cartwheel, dive cartwheel.

Handspring front somersault—A dynamic and fast front handspring that pushes the gymnast into a fast flipping somersault.

Spotting: Gymnast must be able to "punch" out of a handspring first. The spot must come as the feet touch the floor. One hand is on the stomach, other on the shoulder. Holding on to the shoulder is important to prevent over-rotation.

Roundoff-somersault—Eliminating the flip flop, an immediate somersault from the roundoff.

Spotting: Spot as a somersault, but remember to move in after the roundoff.

Roundoff flip flop back somersault tuck

Spotting: If the spotter has to spot the roundoff and flip flop, the gymnast is not ready for the back somersault. As the feet come down on the flip flop, the spotter moves into the back and as the gymnast lifts off the spotter already has his arm around and is lifting. Spotting the landing is equally important, and a spot should be under the stomach lifting, in case the gymnast is under-rotated. The other hand should be grasping the arm to prevent over rotation.

Russian lift front somersault—Arm swing down and up the back at the point of takeoff.

Spotting: When learning, gymnast should not swing arms down but rather start with the arms at the side and swing back. The down lift timing takes longer to learn than the skill. Spot on the back after skill is initiated.

Back pike somersault—A roll over the head in a pike position.
Spotting: Same as a back somersault.

Back straddle somersault—A roll over the head in a pike straddle position.
Spotting: Same.

Cartwheel/layout side—Same as cartwheel dive cartwheel but faster, and no hands on the 2nd cartwheel.
Spotting: Same as aerial cartwheel.

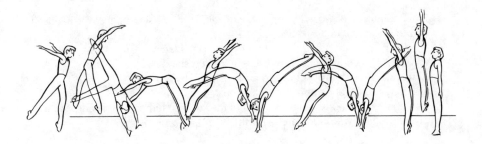

Tumbling and Floor Exercise Progression (Men)

Tumbling and floor exercise activity should start with flexibility work, like the six exercises listed here. These should be done in a smooth, flowing manner.

1. Running for a general overall warm-up.
2. Trunk rotation, forward, backward, right and left sideward, and in a circular movement in both directions.
3. Straddle (side split) in a sitting or standing position.
4. Splits, both right and left.
5. "Pretzel" bend, supine position: Raise legs and bring them up, bent or straight, and touch toes to the mat overhead.
6. Bridge, supine position: Bend the knees and place feet flat on mat and hands on mat by ears with thumbs pointing inward. Rock back and forth.

Skills are presented below in families. They are rated from 1 through 4 on the basis of difficulty, with a 4 rating being the most difficult. If the skill is difficult to perform but is low in danger, it is rated less high than it might be.

Forward Rolls and Variations
1. Roll tucked with or without grasping knees (1).
2. Roll, coming to stand with one leg straight and the other bent (1).
3. Roll to straddled stand (1).
4. Roll from a scale position. Place hands on mat and roll (1) or roll without hands (1+).
5. Roll in a piked position and rise to stand, piked (1+).
6. Headstand, roll out to stand (1).
7. Handstand, roll out to stand (2).
8. Dive roll from a run and hurdle (3). Start the dive from a stand and gradually add steps and a hurdle until the dive is done from a run. At a more advanced level the gymnast can add an obstacle from one and a half to three feet high, such as a padded piece of equipment or another gymnast forming a bridge.
9. Front somersault (3+).

Backward Rolls and Variations
1. From stand, roll tucked (1).
2. Roll backward over one shoulder, placing knee down on the mat. Extend other leg upward and hold a knee scale (1). (This is a good preparation for a fishflop, see 7 below.)

3. From stand, sit down with legs straight (piked) and using hands overhead on mat to push, rise to a piked stand (1+).
4. Sit down in a straddled, straight-leg position, placing hands down between legs, close to body, roll and rise to a straddled stand (1+).
5. Roll and extend body and rise to a headstand (1+).
6. Roll and extend body and rise to a handstand (1+).
7. Roll and extend body, rolling over shoulder or face turned to side and end in a prone position with body arched (fishflop) (2).

Cartwheels and Variations
1. Cartwheel (1).
2. One-handed cartwheel (1+).
3. Roundoff (1+).
4. Run, skip step, diving cartwheel, one handed or two handed (2).
5. Cartwheel to split (1+).
6. Butterfly (2).
7. Aerial cartwheel (3).
8. Side somersault from cartwheel (3+).
9. Roundoff, side somersault (3+).

Balancing
1. Squat headstand (frog headstand) (1).
2. Squat stand (frog stand) (1).
3. Headstand from a tuck, pike or straddle start (1+).
4. Forearm headstand (1+).
5. Forearmstand (1+).
6. Handstand, kick up or press up. (2).

There are several ways to kick to a handstand and many ways to press to one. These slightly add to the difficulty of the skill. There are many ways to recover from a handstand (tuck, pike, straddle down, and the like or bridge out, walkover out, and the like) which add to the difficulty.

Bridging and Front Over
1. Bridge (1).
2. Bridge, extend one leg (1).
3. Bridge, dance (1).
4. Bridge, inside out (1).
5. Headstand, bridgeover (1+).
6. Limberover (2).
7. Kipup or neckspring (2).
8. Headspring, from two-foot takeoff (2).
9. Front walkover (2).
10. Front handspring (2+).
11. Tinsica (2+).
12. One-handed, front walkover (2+).
13. Diving, front walkover (2+).
14. Diving, one-handed, front walkover (2+).
15. Front mounter from handspring (3).

Back Over

1. Backbend, from stand (1+).
2. Backbend and up (1+).
3. Backbend, kickover (2).
4. Back walkover (2).
5. Back limberover (2).
6. One-handed, back walkover (2+).
7. Valdez (2+).
8. Back walkover, straddle through (2+).
9. Back walkover, split through (2±).
10. Back handspring (3).
11. Arabian dive from roundoff or back handspring (3).
12. Back somersault (3+).
13. Arabian mounter (3).
14. Arabian front somersault (4).

Principles for Determining Difficulty. Rolling forward and backward is relatively easy since the body is bent and close to the mat. As the body is raised and extended, as in a handstand or handspring, greater flexibility, strength, and coordination are required by the gymnast and proper spotting by the coach.

When the body is rotated around the lateral axis—as in somersaults or aerials, front, back, or side—great skill is required by the performer, and by the coach when he assists.

Some stunts done in series tend to cause vertigo, and for that reason get an extra rating in difficulty. A series of back or front rolls is an example.

A series of front or back handsprings does increase the difficulty, especially the back handsprings. A roundoff preceding a back handspring or somersault adds to difficulty. A front handspring or tinsica preceding a front somersault adds to difficulty.

Alternating handsprings and somersaults, whether they be front or back, add greatly to the difficulty. A series of bounders (front or back somersaults) are all extremely difficult.

Adding rotations around the long axis (twists) results in extreme difficulty.

Vaulting: Areas of Concern

Vaulting can, and should, be one of the first activities in a gymnastic program. The only prerequisite is a knowledge of basic tumbling. Because vaulting takes less strength of the upper body in comparison with other activities, it can be taught to young boys and girls. Some older boys who lack the upper body strength to be successful in other men's events may do quite well in vaulting.

Of major concern in vaulting is a *mastery of basic movements:* running, jumping, landing, recovery from falls, and basic tumbling movements such as somersaults and rolls. These should be prerequisites for vaulting instruction—no matter how impatient students may be to move on. A track coach can be consulted for help with correct arm and leg action in running. The temptation to over-spot should be avoided, since students get a false sense of security if spotters try to make up for their weaknesses in basic movements.

An intelligent *progression* in teaching is essential. Make sure that students have skills equal to the task. It is like buying insurance to have students overlearn fundamental vaults.

Spotting is especialy important for vaulting. In other events, the dismount usually needs the most careful spotting. In vaulting, every stunt is a dismount. Because there is more horizontal movement in vaulting than in most events, the spotter must learn to move with the performer. Students must practice spotting easy vaults in order to be able to successfully spot difficult vaults.

A large and reasonably *thick mat area* must be provided for the landing. Double thickness mats or special soft landing mats should be used during the learning process. *Board surface* should be checked constantly for non-slip quality.

Because the event requires a fast run, it is important to keep the *approach area clear.* Students working in other events close by must be cautioned to stay out of the vaulting area. Keep bouncing balls out of the area and remove other hazardous objects from around the landing area.

Safety Tips for Instructors and Coaches

1. Make sure that approach area is free of obstructions and traffic, that hazardous building elements are padded, and that the running surface is level and provides good traction (padding is recommended). A smooth, consistent approach run is very important.
2. Check board for position appropriate to type of vault and gymnast's level of proficiency; alse be sure the surface is non-slip and parts are in proper condition.
3. Be sure the horse is securely set at proper height, that mats are ample and properly placed, and that chalk is properly used. (Horse height and selection of mats should be based on gymnast's level of proficiency.)
4. Require mastery of basic skills—running, jumping, landing—before vaulting instruction. Students should be cautioned about the importance of eye contact with the board during the run and then with the horse at point of intended contact during the hurdle. Insist that gymnasts keep eyes open at all times.
5. Make sure there are enough spotters, properly positioned, to help the gymnast in reaching and getting away from the horse safely and in landing without excessive impact.
6. Be sure there is effective communication between spotter and gymnast so that each will know exactly what to expect (nature of vault, type of spot, etc.).
7. In women's vaulting, alert gymnasts and spotters to the importance of making hand contact with the proper area of the horse, toward the approach side and rounded top edge (not on the top flat surface), in order to minimize the possibility of slipping.
8. In teaching post-flights and landings, alert gymnasts and spotters to the extreme hazards of over-rotation, because of the potential for "whiplike" injury to the upper body. Spotters should be alert to a highly angled pre-flight contact, as well as tucking during post-flight, because of danger of over-rotation. In landing, feet should make contact with mats in front of the body and center of gravity, with body extended and knees flexed for absorption of landing shock. Spotter can assist in landing by stabilizing the gymnast's lower back to help prevent over-rotation.

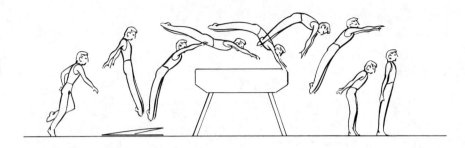

Vaulting Progression (Men or Women)

In other gymnastic activities, as a student becomes more skilled he or she progresses to new skills that are more difficult. In vaulting, however, the more proficient gymnasts perform most of the same vaults that are taught to beginners. The difficulty of the vaults is increased by raising the height of the horse, by executing the vaults in a more difficult manner (layout preflight rather than bent-hips preflight) or, for men, by using a longhorse instead of a crosshorse.

In the teaching progression, crosshorse vaulting should come before longhorse vaulting. Women, of course, vault only over the crosshorse. A good learning technique for some women's vaults, however, is to stand on the near end of a longhorse and practice the after flight phase by placing the hands on the far end and kicking into the postflight.

Another common practice in the teaching progression is to lower the height of the horse, whether it be a crosshorse or a longhorse. A low horse eliminates some of the learner's hesitation in trying a new vault, also makes it easier to spot the performer. Horses should definitely be lowered for children as they are learning to vault. Shoulder height is a rough guide for selecting an appropriate height for boys, while chest height is about right for girls. During the learning process for most vaults, it is wise to lower the horse still more, specifically three to six inches below the usual height used for the particular age level or skill level.

Preliminary Skills or Drills. Practicing the approach and takeoff from the board without the horse is a wise preliminary procedure. In fact, the approach, hurdle, and takeoff can be practiced without a board at first, although this omission is not absolutely necessary in the progression. The vaulter can jump off the board to a self-controlled balanced landing, or can lean forward on the takeoff into the hands of a spotter who supports the hips or ribcage in the air and helps control the landing.

As another lead-up to vaulting, certain skills can be practiced from the takeoff board to the mat. This is more fun than just practicing the approach, hurdle, takeoff, and landing repeatedly without any variations. Some suggestions are:

1. Straight body jump*
2. Arched jump
3. Tuck jump

---

*This can be combined with a variety of arm movements or clapping once, twice, or three times in the air. Clapping can be done in front of the body, behind the body, or over the head.

4. Straddle jump (or straddle over another student)
5. Pike jump
6. Straddle toe touch
7. Half pirouette
8. Full pirouette
9. Pike, arch, pike

Another drill is to dive from the takeoff board into a special mat or from the board over a horse into a special mat. These drills should not be used too early in the progression, however, as they are fairly difficult and need careful supervision. They are best used as a technique for improving layout vaults or vaults in which the feet go over the head in a circular motion, such as head springs, cartwheels and hand springs.

Spotting. Spotters can be placed on the board side of the horse or on the landing side. The preflight spotter is primarily used to assist—that is, to aid the learner in lifting the hips or in attaining rotation (heel lift). This spotter must be alert, however, in case the vaulter fails to pass over the horse and drops back to the floor on the takeoff side. In such cases this spotter becomes a safety spotter and lowers the performer to the floor or at least supports the vaulter as he or she drops back to the feet.

The spotter on the landing side is there primarily for safety purposes, to see that the vaulter lands safely on the feet. For beginning vaulters, the spotter must stand very close to the horse and only slightly to the side of the hand placement zone. The spotter must make contact with the vaulter about the time the vaulter's hands contact the horse, and this contact must be maintained until the spotter is sure that the vaulter will complete the vault in a balanced landing on the feet. For more advanced vaulters that have a long and high afterflight the spotters cannot make early contact but must station themselves at the landing area and be ready to assist as necessary by providing extra rotation or by preventing overrotation. The spotters must be agile and be able to move with the postflight. Even with beginning vaulters, the landing is often some distance from where the spotter makes first-hand contact. The spotter usually moves with the vaulter by taking a large sideward step or several sideward sliding steps.

Progression of Vaulting Skills, Elementary to High Intermediate

Key: E   Elementary   R   Recommended
      I   Intermediate   M   Absolute Must
      HI High Intermediate

	VAULTS	Cross Horse	Dif.	Long Horse Far End	Dif.	Near End	Dif.
1	Squat on jump off straight body	M	E				
2	Squat on jump off with tuck	R	E				
3	Squat on jump off with straddle	R	E				
4	Squat on jump off with pike	R	E				
5	Squat on jump off with straddle and pike	R	E				
6	Squat on jump off with ½ pirouette	R	E				
7	Squat on jump off with full pirouette	R	E				
8	Roll on jump off					R	E
9	Squat, bent hip	M	E	M	E	M	I
10	Rear	R	E				
11	Front, bent hips (face)	M	E				
12	Flank, bent hips (side)	R	E				
13	Straddle, bent hips	M	E	M	E	M	I
14	Wolf	R	E				
15	Courage (knees on jump off)	R	E				
16	Neckspring	R	E				
17	Headspring	M	E	M	I		
18	Front, high straight body	M	E				
19	Stoop, bent hips	M	E				
20	Flank, straight body	R	E				
21	Squat on straddle off			R	E		
22	Squat on squat off			R	E		
23	Squat on stoop off			R	E		
24	Squat on headspring off			R	E		
25	Squat on cartwheel off			R	E		
26	Squat on handspring off			R	E		
27	Roll on bent armspring off			R	E		
28	Squat with ½ turn	R	I	R	I	R	HI
29	Straddle with ½ turn	R	I	R	I	R	HI
30	Stoop with ½ turn	R	I	R	I	R	HI
31	Thief	R	I				
32	Scissors, bent hips			R	I	R	HI
33	Sheep	R	I	R	I	R	HI
34	Flank with ½ or ¾ turn	R	I				
35	Squat on front salto off			R	I		

36	Layout squat	M	HI	M	HI	M	HI
37	Layout straddle	M	HI	M	HI	M	HI
38	Layout squat—stoop					R	HI
39	Layout stoop	M	HI	M	HI	M	HI
40	Front, high, with ½ turn	R	HI				
41	Handstand ¼ turn to cartwheel (and ¼ turn)	R	HI	R	HI		
42	Handstand ¼ turn to front vault	R	HI	R	HI		
43	Hecht	M	HI	M	HI	M	HI
44	Layout scissors			R	HI	R	HI
45	Cartwheel with ¼ turn outward	M	HI	M	HI		
46	Handstand squat off	R	HI				
47	Handstand straddle off	R	Hi				
48	Handstand stoop off	R	HI				
49	Handspring	M	HI	M	HI	M	HI
50	Yamashita	M	HI	M	HI	M	HI

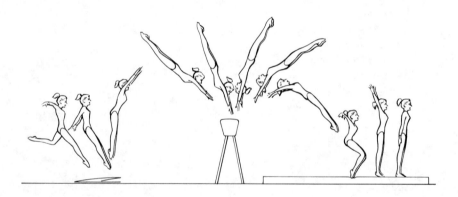

Vaulting Progression (Women)

This outline only partially reflects the various possible progressions in vaulting instruction for women. The following can be hazards: any landing, catching feet on the horse during certain vaults, hands slipping from the horse, missing the horse with hands altogether, and slipping from the board. All vaulting apparatus should be checked and prepared for effective and safe use. An instructor should always be near the apparatus.

Running Development (elements)

1. Effective arm motions
2. Effective leg usages
3. Arm and leg synchronization

4. Running on the balls of feet
5. Accurate relative stride length according to physical growth and development
6. Proper head position
7. Developing a positive mental attitude
8. Consultation with running experts for running methods
9. Exercises to strengthen body parts involved
10. Build-up of run till a secure distance is obtained
11. Measuring run for accuracy
12. Timing the run for consistency
13. Coordinating run and hurdle
14. Effective eye-board coordination upon approach

Hurdle Development and Board Usage (instructions)

1. Stand on board and bounce several times on balls of feet to become aware of board action.
2. Jump on board, rebound off to landing mat.
3. Jump from floor to board (one step), bringing both feet together on board, rebound to board.
4. From a three-step run, jump from floor to floor in low-short quick action, using effective arm and leg action.
5. From a three-step run jump from floor to the board in a low-shortquick action, depress the board, and repulse to the landing mat.
6. Be aware of effective arm usage from floor to board.

Landing Skill Development (instructions)

1. Jump from floor to floor in a hopping manner, flexing legs on the down part of the hop, with a slight space between the feet and a slight bend of the hips, with the buttocks tucked under in body alignment. Balls of feet should contact the floor first. Six to eight inches is suggested as the best distance between feet in landing from a vault.
2. Jump from board to floor and stress body tightness upon repulsion.
3. Start to graduate height following the same procedures suggested above.
4. Learn effective techniques for rolling forward or backward to be used on incorrect landing. On any rolls, always support body weight on hands and not on neck or head.
5. Avoid side landings of any kind.

Body Position for Pre-flight, Repulsion and After-flight Development

1. Develop flight and on-horse awareness through preparatory exercises which include: body tightness, proper posture, flight angles.
2. Develop consistency and kinesthetic awareness.
3. Build skill progression from exercises to floor drills to graduated heights to final vault execution. Here is a checklist:

Skill	Difficulty	Spotting
Squat	Beg.	Easy
Flank	Beg.	Easy

Wolk	Beg.	Easy
Straddle	Beg.	Easy
Stoop	Beg.	Easy
Horizontal Squat	Int.	Int.
Horizontal Straddle	Int.	Int.
Layout Squat	Diff.	Diff.
Layout Straddle	Diff.	Diff.
Layout Stoop	Diff.	Diff.
Handspring	Adv.	Adv.

4. Be sure the horse *always* is cleared by a safe distance.

Pommel Horse: Areas of Concern

Although the pommel horse offers fewer chances for major injury than other men's activities, it is not immune to hazards. Painful bruises, strains, or scrapes are not uncommon, and serious sprains or fractures are possible.

Discussion and practice of *specific falling recovery movements* should be a prerequisite for pommel horse training, because falling from the horse differs in significant ways from other gymnastic falls. For one thing, a gymnast may have trouble keeping aware of his center of gravity during a pommel horse movement. For another, the prime safety rule in a fall is to hold on to the horse in any way possible—with one or two hands—until some portion of the body has made contact with the mat.

Structured workout programs with clear progressions are important for two reasons. One is the difficulty of both hand and belt spotting in pommel horse activities. The other is that the apparent relative safety of the horse can lead gymnasts into over-ambition or under-seriousness. A game like follow-the-leader combines an ego trip with horse play, often with unfortunate results.

Proper matting and protective gymnastic clothing are essential, especially to avoid leg injuries. Base filler mats should be ample and correctly placed, and gymnasts should be given level surfaces for working and dismounting.

Safety Tips for Instructors and Coaches

1. Check horse for appropriate adjustments and proper functioning before and periodically during the activity. Make sure the height is appropriate for the gymnasts' level of proficiency, that pommels are tightened, and that locking mechanisms are secure.
2. Check mats for adequacy and proper arrangement before and throughout the activity.
3. Make sure gymnasts have mastered mounting and falling recovery movements. Sprains and jamming of fingers and thumbs can be avoided by placing hands on the pommels or body of the horse before mounting (as opposed to jumping up and then grabbing onto the horse).
4. Make sure gymnasts are wearing proper gymnastic clothing as protection against bumps and scrapes.

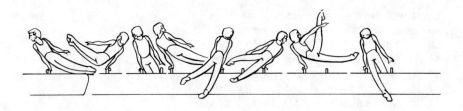

Pommel Horse Progression (Men)

The progressions outlined here need not be followed to the letter. Note also that many lead-up skill possibilities have been omitted because pommel horse sequences are almost limitless. The following progressions comprise a safe guide to learning basic skills, assuming the apparatus is stable and adequate matting is provided.

All of the drills and skills listed may be considered *elementary* except where noted as intermediate (Int.).

1. Front Support
2. Rear Support
3. Front Support—Left Leg Forward—Left Leg Back
4. Repeat 3 with Right Leg
5. Rear Support—Left Leg Back—Left Leg Forward
6. Repeat 5 with Right Leg
7. Stride Support with Left Leg Forward—Swing Left Leg Right Under Right Hand to Front Support—Repeat in Opposite Position
8. Stride Support with Left Leg Forward—Swing Right Leg Forward Under Left Hand and Repeat in Reverse
9. Front Support—Right Leg Forward Under Left Hand
10. Repeat 9 with Left Leg Under Right Hand
11. Rear Support—Right Leg Back Under Left Hand
12. Repeat 11—Left Leg Back Under Right Hand
13. Single Leg Side Travel from Middle to End
14. Single Leg Side Travel from End to Middle
15. Single Leg Side Travel with Back Scissor to End
16. Front Support—Swing Right Leg Forward Under Left Hand and Right Hand in Series of Three
17. Repeat 16 to Opposite Side
18. Rear Support—Swing Left Leg Back Under Right Hand and Left Hand to Rear Support—Repeat Three Times
19. Front Support—Swing Both Legs Under Left Hand to Rear Support
20. Repeat 19 to Opposite Side
21. Rear Support—Swing Both Legs Under Right Hand to Front Support
22. Repeat 21 to Opposite Side
23. Feint to Half Circle
24. Repeat 23 to Opposite Side
25. Back Scissor from Stride Support
26. Repeat in Opposite Direction
27. Front Scissor from Stride Support

28. Repeat in Opposite Direction
29. Jump into Half Circle from Stand
30. *Int.* Jump or Feint into One or More Circles
31. *Int.* Stride Support—Swing Rear Forward into Circle (in Best Circle Direction)
32. *Int.* Stride Support—Swing Forward Leg Back into Circle (Best Circle Direction)
33. *Int.* Kehre in Mount (Hand Spot Beginners)
34. *Int.* Moore (Czeck) Mount
35. *Int.* Circles on Croup and Neck of Horse
36. *Int.* Side Travel from Circles (Travel Down)
37. Double Rear Dismount from Feint
38. Triple Rear Dismount from Feint
39. *Int.* Side Travel Dismount from Circles
40. *Int.* Kehre Out Dismount from Circles

Still Rings: Areas of Concern

Success and safety on the rings depend on the *simultaneous development of strength and skill.* Even the correct execution of skills in this activity places great stress on all of the structures of the upper body, particularly the shoulder joints. Incorrect execution can injure the joints of the strongest gymnast. Therefore, if there is emphasis on correct technique in the earliest stages of training, injuries are less likely to occur at later stages of development.

In working with gymnasts at the beginning level the *first skills should be presented with the rings at shoulder height.* These skills require some degree of strength, balance, flexibility, and kinesthetic awareness. They should be attempted under the direction of a certified instructor and a knowledgable spotter. There should be ample mats in place also.

Dismounts require special training. All somersaults, twisting somersaults, double somersaults, and twisting double somersaults are movements best taught on a trampoline using a belt suspended from overhead. Progression in learning these movements is available from manufacturers. When doing these movements on the rings, it is best to use an overhead belt. After the gymnast has done the skill many times he should proceed to do it with hand spotting and ample mats. Some facilities have pits filled with foam and some use 12-inch foam mats. However, care must be taken to avoid knee and ankle injuries when landing on soft surfaces.

Swinging movements should be introduced with extreme care because of the strain they put on the upper body and also because of the danger of falls. A gymnast should be able to close his hand around the ring, and should know exactly how high a swing is safe for his strength and skill. All skills done with great swing must be treated with respect because the gymnast is likely to lose his grip at the moment of greatest speed. This usually occurs as the gymnast is just past the vertical hang ascending forward or backward. If his hands pull off at this moment, he leaves the rings in a low trajectory with his body rotating in an uncontrolled manner. Every attempt must be made to avoid this type of fall, as it is the most dangerous. It is almost impossible to spot, and the best prevention is in mastery of the technique of swinging. Ample mats are vitally important.

In ring activities, especially swinging, *the condition of the hands is of great importance.* Gymnastic chalk should always be readily available, and the instructor/coach should check hand guards and taping (if any). When a gymnast has serious lacerations on his hands, he should be discouraged from swinging. Recently some gymnasts have started wearing a dowel under or built into the hand grip; the use of such devices should be confined to advanced work after consultation with the instructor/coach, as noted in Chapter 6.

Most important is the judgment of a competent coach, who not only guides the long range development by presenting the proper progression, but who also makes the decisions of the moment regarding the direction and duration of daily training.

Safety Tips for Instructors and Coaches

1. Check apparatus and mats before and throughout the activity. Make sure cables, turnbuckles, swivels, fittings, straps, and rings themselves are in good working condition.
2. Make sure gymnasts are physically prepared. A gymnast should be able to close his hand around the ring, and should be told exactly what skills he has the strength to perform—especially how high a swing is safe for him.
3. Check condition of gymnasts' hands, and be sure chalk is used properly.
4. Use low rings for beginning or new skills.
5. Introduce swinging movements carefully, noting danger of slipping off rings caused by improper arm position (swinging with bent arms).
6. Use enough spotters, properly positioned. Generally a spotter is directly in line with the vertical hang of the rings. Use of a spotting platform can be advantageous in teaching new or advanced skills. Do not hesitate to use extra spotters when teaching new or advanced skills, especially if swinging is involved.
7. Train spotters to spot above the center of gravity of the gymnast's body when it is in free position in the air, and to avoid grabbing below the hips.
8. In teaching dismounts, especially after swings, be sure the spotter is experienced in assisting with each particular dismount. Do not hesitate to use special mats and overhead belts.

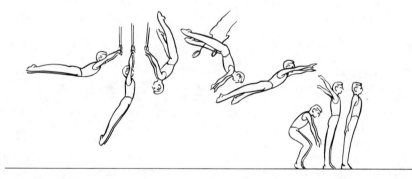

Still Rings Progression (Men)

The first positions to be mastered are:
From a stand turn rearways to

1. inverted squat hang—return to stand;

2. inverted piked hang—return to stand;
3. hang rearways—return to stand;
4. inverted hang with hips stretched (slightly arched back)—return to stand.

Then all of these positions should be combined into one routine and finished with a bent arms hang (hands at chest) prior to dismounting. Many repetitions of this routine, done slowly with control and good form, prepare the musculo-skeletal system and the nervous system for more advanced movements.

When the student demonstrates both mental and physical readiness, it is time to introduce the inlocate and dislocate. With the rings at shoulder height, inward and outward rotation of the rings can be repeated many times.

Inlocate Jump and, while turning forward, rotate the arms inwardly, finishing in an inverted piked hang.

Dislocate Turn backward slowly to a stand, then rotate the arms outwardly, moving from a hang stand rearways to a regular stand.

By repeating these movements many times the gymnast lays a foundation for the inlocate from a swing and the dislocate from a piked hang. It is also prudent to begin support work with the rings shoulder high so that the novice will not fall through the rings in a manner which would increase stress on shoulder, elbow, or wrist joints. When the rings are low and the participant falls through the rings, the feet hit the ground first, avoiding considerable force. Exercises to build strength and skill are

1. Straight arm support position—hold 10 seconds.
2. Dips—from bent arm support to straight arm support.
3. Straight arm support in squat and/or piked position, thighs in horizontal plane.
4. From a support turn slowly forward to a piked hang—spotter has hand under gymnast's upper back.
5. Attempt shoulder stand balance—spotter slows descent.
6. Attempt handstand—spotter slows descent. (A foam pad should be in place under the rings.)
7. Rings at reach high—with high (false) grip pull-push to straight arm support.

With the rings in a jump high position the novice gymnast should learn to swing forward and backward. The swing should be done with straight arms, with the feet leading in a natural, rhythmical manner. Once the swing is done smoothly, the performer should swing to a piked inverted hang. Best results are attained by having students take short turns, followed by short rests. Repetition builds strength and skill, but fatigue generates increased risk of losing grips on the rings as well as poor technique. As the gymnast displays greater ability to swing, the basic swing skills can be learned. The first skill to attempt is the inlocate. Since the gymnast has already done many with the rings low, it is easy to accomplish when his backward swing gives him a feeling of weightlessness, and when his instructor, at the appropriate moment, lifts the abdomen with one hand and cradles the back of the neck with the other.

The dislocate should be taught with the rings at the head high position so that the instructor can cushion the descent of the gymnast emphasizing the complete outward rotation of the arms before the body descends. When taking the gymnast to the high rings, great care must be taken in spotting the gymnast, not only as he descends, but especially as his body passes the vertical and ascends. One hand can be on the abdomen and one hand on the upper back as the performer's body ascends. The inlocate from swing and the dislocate from piked hang are skills to be mastered before more difficult swinging skills are attempted. The aforementioned movements provide the foundation for the development of higher value movements. Although individual differences exist among participants, there is universal agreement that skills should be taught in an order which progresses from the simple to the more difficult. If the proper progression is followed, risk of injury is minimized.

Listed below are skills in an approximate order of difficulty and risk with safety factors mentioned.

1. From piked hang kip to support. Rings should be head high. Spot under thighs and buttocks.
2. Uprise (stemme) to support on rear swing. Rings jump high position. Spot front of thighs at knees as support position is reached.
3. Uprise to support on forward swing. Rings jump high. Spot legs in case gymnast falls through with an arm behind his back.
4. From swing straddle cut dismount backwards. Rings jump high. Spot with one hand on chest and one on back to prevent under- and over-rotation.
5. From piked inverted hang straddle cut dismount forward. Rings head high. Spot one hand behind neck, one under arm.
6. Kip backward to support. Rings head high. Spot one hand on chest, one on thigh.
7. Kip backward to shoulderstand. Rings head high. Have hand follow lower back in order to slow descent in case of forward fall.
8. Kip backward to handstand. Same as above, but have extra mat to cushion heels in case of forward fall.
9. Back uprise to handstand. Have gymnast build swing progressively to prevent the jerky motion which can cause loss of grip.
10. From shoulderstand and from handstand fall forward to back uprise. Same as above, but be ready to spot chest as gymnast ascends.
11. Forward giant swing. Same as above.
12. Backward giant swing. Spot in same manner as dislocate but expect many times the force. If possible spot with an overhead belt, being aware of how difficult it is to get the slack out of the lines quickly. Have thick mats in place.

Balance Beam: Areas of Concern

Balance beam essentially involves skills learned in tumbling and dance. Thus, beam progressions often involve, not the original learning of the skill, but rather adjustments for performing the skill on a narrow, straight line several feet above the ground.

Perhaps the cardinal rule for balance beam is that the *high beam is not the place for learning new skills*. The gymnast should first learn the skill at the floor level. After demonstrating her ability to consistently perform the skill on a straight line, the gymnast should then move to a low beam where the skill should be mastered prior to moving to the higher beams. The low training beam, preferably, should be low enough that the gymnast can straddle the beam with both feet on the floor without touching the beam. If a low beam is not available, mats can be placed under the beam to achieve the same effect. The use of padded low beams and/or mats piled along side the beam to a point level with its top surface is also highly recommended.

During the initial learning stages, the instructor should provide the gymnast with *spotting assistance* until the gymnast has satisfactorily demonstrated both the mental and physical preparation to consistently perform the skill safely. Even during the intermediate stages of learning the skill, the instructor should be positioned in a state of readiness to help the gymnast should such assistance become necessary.

It is possible to develop skills safely on the high balance beam without physically spotting the gymnast. However, this approach requires a commitment on the part of both the coach and the gymnast to a program of careful, time-consuming, painstaking preparation. The gymnast's skills must be developed carefully by demonstrating mastery of the skills at each level of preparation, starting first on the floor level and progressing through many levels of beam heights until the skill is finally performed on the high beam. This technique takes many, many hours of preparation for each skill. A supervising instructor/coach may decide to omit some levels of beam heights from a balance beam progression, but should insist on *mastery of all skills at the floor level.*

Because the gymnast is typically performing skills which she has already mastered on the floor, the balance beam can often appear deceptively safe. Running and skipping on the beam may seem relatively safe, but a small wobble or slip on the high beam can produce a fall with consequences as serious as if the fall had been produced by a misstep on an advanced skill. Thus, the use of low beams, particularly with younger children, is highly recommended. *Learning to fall properly, or to recover from a fall, should accompany every skill.*

Safety Tips for Instructors and Coaches

1. Make sure the apparatus is secure and level, and that appropriate mats are in place.
2. Check beam surface periodically. Replace tops if loose, worn, ragged, or slippery. Resurface wood tops if pitted, worn, or in poor condition. Replace excessively warped wood beams.
3. Use low beams and/or additional mats when teaching new skills and dismounts.
4. Be sure gymnasts use proper footwear to provide necessary traction.
5. Insist on mastery of all skills at floor level before they are tried on the beam.
6. Provide adequate spotting for all new skills on the beam, especially dismounts, which present more hazards than unintended contact with the beam. Use safety belts when needed for effective spotting, plus additional mats under beginning conditions.
7. Insist on mastery of proper learning methods and progressions before introduction of aerial skills, which are especially hazardous without thorough preparation. Extreme safety precautions should be exercised during all training and practice of aerial skills.

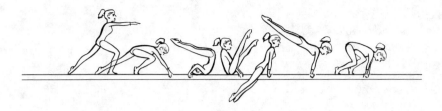

Balance Beam Progression (Women)

Key: *Importance*

R—recommended
HR—highly recommended
M—absolute must

Difficulty

LB—low beginning
B—beginning
HB—high beginning
LI—low intermediate
I—intermediate
HI—high intermediate
A—advanced

Mounts

Use Beat Board Perpendicular to side of the Beam

Jump to front support	R	LB
Jump to squat, on hand support	R	B
Jump to ½ straddle hand support (lunge)	R	B
Jump to straddle on hand support	R	B
Jump to squat through hand support	R	HB
Jump to stoop through hand support	R	LI
Jump to straddle through hand support	R	HB
Jump to squat—no hand support	R	HI-A
Jump to ½ straddle (lunge) no hand support	R	HI-A
Jump to straddle no hand support	R	HI-A

Use Beat Board Diagonal to Beam

Jump to side seat or near side	R	LB
Jump hitch kick over & side seat on far side	HR	LB
Jump hitch kick over ½ turn side seat on far side	R	B
Run on to squat position using 1 hand support	HR	B
Run on to stand using momentum hand support	R	HB
Run on to squat using momentum no hand support	R	I
Run on to stand using momentum no hand support	R	HI
Run to hand support to forward roll on	R	I

Using Beat Board Perpendicular to end of Beam

Jump to hand support forward roll	R	I
Hand support push off to squat on	R	I
No hand support run to squat on	R	HI
No hand support run to squat on stand scale ½ turn to scale	R	A

Rolls

Forward Shoulder	R	LB
Forward Over the Head	M	B
No-Hand Roll	R	I
Backward Over the Shoulder	R	LB
Backward Over the Head	HR	HB
Back Extension	R	HI
English Handstand Roll Down	R	HI

Handstands

Side Handstand Straddle Down	HR	I
Side Handstand Straddle Through	HR	HI
Handstand Pirouette	HR	HI
Balance Side Handstand	HR	HI
Balance English Handstand	HR	HI

Wheels

Two-Arm Cartwheel	HR	I
One-Arm Cartwheel (near & far)	R	HI
Back Walkover	HR	I
Back Walkover to Handstand	R	I
Back Walkover Switch	R	I
Front Walkover	HR	HI
Front Walkover Switch Leg	R	HI
Front Walkover Stag	R	HI
Back Tinsica	R	HI
Front Tinsica	R	HI
Back Handspring	HR	HI
Front Handspring Step-out	HR	HI
One-Arm Back Walkover	R	HI
One-Arm Front Walkover	R	HI

Dismounts

Jump	R	LB
Knee Scale	R	LB
V Sit	R	LB
Roundoff (cartwheel not recommended)	HR	B
Roundoff One Arm	R	HB
Cartwheel ¼ turn out (land facing away from beam)	R	I
Handstand Underbalance	R	HB
Handstand ¼ Turn	HR	LI
Front Handspring Off End	R	I
Side Aerial	R	HI(A)
Front Aerial	R	HI(A)
Back Somi	HR	HI
Front Somi	HR	HI(A)

Locomotive Moves

Walk forward, sideways, backward	M	LB
Walk forward, sideways, backward on halftoe	M	B
Dip Step	HR	B
Step Kick	HR	B
Waltz Step (Step Close Step)	HR	B
Waltz Step (Down UP UP)	HR	B
Run	M	HB
Chasse	M	HB

Hops and Leaps

Step Hop (Skip)	M	HB
Sissone	HR	HB
Two-Foot Jump	HR	HB
Essemble	R	HB
Cat Leap	R	HB
Tuck Jump	HR	LI
Changement	HR	LI
Hitchkick	HR	LI
Leap (grande jete)	M	I

Poses

Knee Scale	R	LB
V Sit	R	LB
Lunge	HR	B
Scale	HR	B
Arabesque	HR	HB
Stork, front scale holding foot	R	B
Half split	R	B
Split	HR	HB

Turns

Two-Foot Toe Turn	M	LB
Squat	R	LB
Swing Forward	HR	B
Swing Backward	HR	B
Lunge High	R	B
Lunge Low	R	HB
Pique	R	HB
Chaine	R	HB
Inward Pirouette (forward)	HR	HB
Outward Pirouette (backward)	HR	HB
Full	M	I

Parallel Bars: Areas of Concern

Proper progression, mastery of basic skills, and curbing of over-enthusiasm are important in parallel bar activities because of the considerable upper body strain and risk of falls. *Low bars should be used for basic or new skills.*

Adequate, properly placed mats are essential. Bases should be covered and uneven surfaces avoided, in order to assure safe landings. *Additional mats should be used in teaching difficult skills.*

Correct spotting is a matter of concern. Normally spotting should be from below the bars and through them, since a spotter's arms above the bars can result in injury to him and the gymnast.

Safety Tips for Instructors and Coaches

1. Check apparatus before and throughout the activity; be sure rails are level, secure, and in good condition. Replace cracked or excessively warped rails and worn parts.
2. Be sure mats are adequate and properly placed to cover bases and to provide a level landing surface. Use additional mats in teaching beginning or difficult skills, especially dismounts.
3. Make sure gymnasts use chalk properly.
4. Adjust the bars according to the gymnast's size, strength, and level of proficiency. Use low bars for teaching new skills, and working on some advanced skills. Move rails closer together for smaller gymnasts.
5. Use enough spotters, properly positioned, for the level of proficiency of the gymnast and the difficulty of the skill. Spotting platforms (e.g., folded mats) and safety belts should be used when needed for effective, and safe spotting.
6. Make sure spotters use safe methods and get help when needed. In normal hand spotting, arms should reach between the bars from below. In general reaching across the bars places the spotter in an accident-prone position.

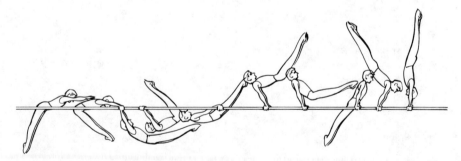

Parallel Bars Progression (Men)

The performer should work up progressively to the listed number of sets and repetitions. This will increase strength, skill, and control and, thus, better prepare the performer to advance to the more difficult skills.

Elementary

1. Modified chin-ups with feet on floor—10 repetitions (reps)

2. From hang, hook legs over bars and climb through—6 reps
3. Jump up to hand support—10 reps
4. Handwalk (penguin)—one length forward and backward
     Spotter: Stands behind performer and holds waist.
5. Hand support hopping—one length forward and backward
     Spotter: Same as for 4.
6. Push-ups on bars—2 sets of 10 reps
7. Straddle leg travels—Length of bars forward and backward twice
8. Straight hand support 180° turn—2 sets of 5 reps
9. Hand support with feet on bars, jump off bars and swing forward to stand on bars in front of hands—3 sets of 5 reps
10. Forward swing to rear vault dismount—5 reps

Elementary—Intermediate

11. Back scissor turn (180°)—2 sets of 3 reps
12. Swing in hand support—2 sets of 10 swings
13. Straight body swings with body reaching the horizontal at both ends of swing—2 sets of 10 swings.
     Note: Perform initially on low parallel bars.
14. With one leg over opposite bar, one leg flank dismount—5 reps
15. From front support on one bar, cast away and return—2 sets of 3 reps
16. Dips—2 sets of 8 reps
17. Pull-ups with feet on bars—2 sets of 10 reps
18. Forearm uprise—2 sets of 5 reps (without swing)
19. Forearm front uprise—2 sets of 3 reps
20. Uprise (without swing) from upper arm—2 sets of 3 reps
21. From hang, skin-the-cat—2 sets of 3 reps
22. Forward swing with ¼ turn into the bar (rear vault ¼ turn)—5 reps
23. Forward turnover mount on end—5 reps
24. Backward turnover mount on end—4 reps
25. Leg push rise to support on end—5 reps
26. Back swing to front vault dismount—5 reps
27. Front uprise—2 sets of 3 reps
     Spotter: Place one hand under legs and the other hand under lower back and help lift when performer pushes down.
28. Back uprise—2 sets of 3 reps
     Spotter: Place one hand on abdomen and the other hand on the thigh and help performer up.
29. From front leaning support, opposite leg and arm balance—2 sets of 3 reps
30. Piked inverted upper arm position whereby the legs are held horizontal over the head—2 sets of 3 reps
31. On end, one leg cut mount—3 sets of 2 reps
     Spotter: Stands behind performer lifting him by the waist.
32. Straddle seat, upper arm forward roll to straddle seat—3 sets of 2 reps
     Note: Perform first on very low parallel bars and with mat over the bars in front of performer. Then use spotter on higher bars.

Intermediate

33. Straddle seat press to upper arm balance ("shoulderstand")— 6 sets of 1 rep
    Note: Perform first on very low parallel bars with mat over bars in front of performer.
    Spotter: Stands to side reaching under bar and places one hand under shoulder and the other hand under back to prevent falling over or through bars.
34. Roll forward from an upper arm balance—2 sets of 2 reps
    Note: Perform first on matted low bars.
    Spotter: Place hands under bars at shoulder and back of performer to slow down roll.
35. Upper arm kip to straddle seat—2 sets of 2 reps
    Spotter: Helps lift performer into kip, thus giving him the feeling of action.
36. Upper arm kip—2 sets of 2 reps
    Spotter: Stands at side and helps lift the performer by placing hand on back under bars which are waist high. Simultaneously, the spotter places the other hand in front of the performer's chest upon the leg thrust in order to prevent any forward fall.
37. One elbow planch with other hand holding onto far bar—6 sets of 1 rep
38. Forward swing to rear vault with half turn inward dismount—3 sets of 2 reps
39. Swing to upper arm balance—6 sets of 1 rep
    Note: The "shoulder" balance is usually arrived at by way of a tucked swing, followed by a piked swing and, finally, a straight body swing.
    Spotter: Same as for press to "shoulder" balance (33).
40. Forward swinging dips—2 sets of 6 reps
41. Backward swinging dips—2 sets of 5 reps
42. Piked backward upper arm roll—5 sets of 1 rep
    Spotting is advisable for beginners.
43. Pull over on one bar—6 sets of 1 rep
44. Straddle leg cut mount on end—6 sets of 1 rep
    Spotter: Stands behind performer lifting him by the waist.
45. From an upper arm balance, sideward fall dismount—5 sets of 1 rep
    Spotter: Stands at side of performer and places one hand under the upper back and the other hand under the legs upon the drop. Proceed to lift performer on the ascent if he needs it.

Perform the above stunts in various sequences before proceeding to the following skills.

Intermediate—Advanced

47. One leg cut in middle of bars
48. Double leg flank cut in middle of bars
49. Double leg straddle cut in middle of bars—3 reps
50. Glide kip in middle of bars
51. Straddle cut dismount from end of bars
    Spotter: Stands in front of performer catching the upper arm as the performer leaves the bars.

52. Extended body back shoulder roll from upper arms
    Use spotter at first.
53. At end of bars facing out, kick up to a handstand. Then, over balance and recover by turning out and landing on feet.
    Note: Competence should first be gained on the floor, then proceed to the low bars before going to the higher bars, where a spotter should be used.
54. From a straight arm support, swing the body from the shoulders increasing the amplitude (opening up the arm-body angle) so that the body approaches a handstand—10 reps
55. Swing to handstand on end
    Spotter: Stands on the same side as the arm that the performer turns out on.
56. Handstand over balance and turn out in middle of bars
    Note: First perform on low bars and use spotter.
57. Handstand lower to upper arm balance and roll over
    Note: First perform on low bars.
58. Forward dip swing stutz (½ turn) to upper arms
59. Forward dip swing stutz to hand support
60. Back uprise straddle cut to hand support
61. From a stand with an inner grip, jump into an underbar cast to upper arm
    Spotter: Stands at side and places both hands under back of performer and lifts performer as needed.
62. Double rear dismount
    Spotter: Stands at side and holds arm the performer will be supported on.
63. Back uprise ½ turn to upper arm
    Spotter: Stands at side and lifts performer as he turns into stunt.
64. Back uprise ½ turn to hand support
    Spotter: Same as 63 except that the spotter must really hold performer up and delay the falling action thus giving the performer more time to turn and complete the stunt before dropping.
65. Wende (Windy) dismount
    Note: First perform from still handstand on end of bars and eventually proceed to mid bars from a swing.
    Spotter: Grasps the arm performer pirouettes on and helps off sideways if necessary.
66. Hollander (handstand pirouette to cartwheel) dismount
    Note: Same progression as the Wende dismount—65.
    Spotter: Stands facing the back side of the performer as he cartwheels off, then reaches for his waist as he descends and controls his drop so that he lands adequately.
67. Handstand forward pirouette
    Note: First perfect on floor, then proceed to low bars with spotter and finally to higher bars with spotter.
68. Swinging forward pirouette
    Note: Initially perform on low bars by kicking to handstand and pirouetting immediately, then proceed to higher bars with a spotter.
69. Forward stutz to upper arm
    Note: First perform on padded bars

70. Stutz to support

> *Note:* First perform on end of bars, then in middle with a spotter.
>
> *Spotter:* Stands on a platform at side of performer and catches body upon ½ turn.

71. Back stutz to straddle seat
72. Back stutz with spotter. Spotting is similar to the forward stutz —70.

Uneven Parallel Bars: Areas of Concern

Proper progression and mastery of basic skills need constant emphasis because of the temptation—on the part of some instructors and coaches as well as gymnasts—to seek the sensational uneven bar skill rather than the artistry of the entire activity. Regular and honest evaluations of progress are essential.

The *condition of the apparatus should be checked constantly,* and the manufacturer's recommended installation, care, and maintenance procedures followed strictly. Specified mats always should be used—plus additional mats when new skills are being learned.

Correct spotting is of vital concern because of the rapid and complex movements in this activity, and because of the dangers to the gymnast and the spotter from spotting errors. The spotter should place himself in a position that allows him/her enough leverage to provide adequate support to the gymnast, and should avoid letting his/her arm get between the gymnast and the bar.

Safety Tips for Instructors and Coaches

1. Make sure the apparatus is designed and installed for necessary stability and safety. For instance, only limited exercises should be permitted when parallel bar conversion units are used, since these have limited stability.
2. Check apparatus before and throughout the activity. Make sure bars themselves and supporting devices (floorplates, cables, turnbuckles, attachments, and locking mechanisms) are in safe condition. Replace unsafe bars and other parts. Check manufacturer's maintenance procedures.
3. Use mats prescribed for competition plus additional mats for safe teaching of new or difficult skills, especially dismounts. Don't skimp on mats!
4. Check condition of gymnast's hands and proper use of chalk.
5. Insist on gymnast's mastery of basic skills and proper progression. Emphasize dangers in shortcuts.
6. Don't hesitate to use additional spotters, or safety mechanics, properly positioned to have the leverage needed for adequate support of the gymnast, particularly for advanced skills. Use folded mats or soft spotting platforms for safety in the event a gymnast collides with them.
7. In spotting low bar skills, try to spot from underneath the bar in order to avoid injury to both gymnast and spotter from having the spotter's arm caught between gymnast and bar.
8. When the gymnast is in motion, spot at the center of gravity or hips for maximum effectiveness. When the gymnast is in the air (free position), spot above the center of gravity or hips to protect head and neck. Spotting uneven bar activities is especially difficult and hazardous because of rotational skills,

constant changes of direction, releases and regress, inversions, grip changes, and movements from one bar to the other.

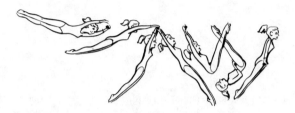

Uneven Parallel Bars Progression (Women)

As in all gymnastic events, uneven bars involve a variety of skills, some closely related to each other while others are markedly different. The skills in the kipping family, for example, are very similar to each other; yet quite different skills are required for seat circles. Therefore, any list of progressions must have a number of branching points where one family of skills can be substituted for another family of skills. A gymnast could start a kip progression or a seat circle progression without one being a prerequisite for the other, although both require that the gymnast be capable of supporting her body weight.

Within each family of skills, a safe progression of movements has been outlined. The families have been arranged in an order of generally increasing difficulty; however, as noted, some skill groups are not prerequisites for others. A back hip circle must be mastered before a cast wrap, yet a glide kip can be taught before or after the gymnast learns a seat circle. Nonetheless, there is some overlap between the progressions outlined within each family of skills.

One important point—although these progressions do represent the consensus of many experienced teachers and coaches of gymnastics, they most certainly are not the only safe progressions which might be used. For those teachers and coaches who are seeking a safe, sane set of progressions for gymnastics, this list represents *one* (but not the only) set of progressions which have been used successfully and safely over many years by many experienced instructors teaching in a wide variety of gymnastic programs. These progressions cover the major basic gymnastic skills, but no attempt has been made to include high-level, advanced skills of extreme difficulty.

Finally, a list of progressions is not a substitute for sound judgment and a safety conscious attitude. The list can, however, provide the serious instructor with a good working tool.

Key:
LB—Low Beginner   R—Recommended
B—Beginner   HR—Highly Recommended
HB—High Beginner   M—Absolute Must
LI—Low Intermediate
I—Intermediate
A—Advanced

Swing Technique

Swing (i.e., pendulum movement) is basic to almost all uneven bar movements. Besides the body awareness which develops as the individual becomes accustomed to the swinging movements, swing drills help develop grip strength, general body tone, self-confidence, and calloused hands, all necessary for more advanced bar work.

Low Bar Swings

1.	Skin-the-cat	R	LB
2.	Monkey swings—hands in overgrip, pump swing	R	LB
	a) ½ turn releasing one hand to mixed grip		
	b) ½ turn releasing one hand at a time to finish in an overgrip		
	c) ½ turn with simultaneous release of both hands to finish in overgrip		
	d) multiple swing, ½ turns without stopping		
3.	Hands and feet swings under the bar	HR	LB
	a) straddle swing		
	1) overgrip		
	2) undergrip		
	b) stoop swing		
	1) overgrip		
	2) undergrip		
4.	Hock swings—hands in overgrip, one leg hooked over low bar	R	LB
	a) simple pump swings		
	b) to stride support above low bar		
	c) from stride support, drop back into hock swing		
5.	Basket swings—hands in overgrip, feet free of bar	HR	B
	a) pike compression		
	1) overgrip		
	2) undergrip		
	b) straddle compression		
	1) overgrip		
	2) undergrip		

6. Glide swings—hands in overgrip   M   B
    a) jump to glide, straddle or stoop
    b) iso-glides—continuous glides in straddle or stoop
    c) glide switch glide—straddle glide, ½ turn, straddle glide

High Bar Swings

1. Hang facing low bar, pump swing legs to low bar   HR   LB
    a) squat on
    b) stoop on
    c) squat over to extended rear support
    d) straddle over to extended rear support
    e) stoop over to extended rear support
2. Long hang swings—overgrip, facing away from low bar   HR   LB
    a) start from hanging position
    b) start from sitting position on low bar
    c) start from squat or standing position on low bar
    d) from sitting position on low bar, swing to overarched position, then straddle or stoop back to sitting position on low bar
3. Beat swings—long hang, squat push off from low bar to wrap in on low bar   HR   B
    Caution—gymnast must be strong enough to maintain her grip on bar, especially on back swing.
4. Stomach whip swings   M   B
    a) from stomach whip position, one hand on high bar in overgrip, one hand on low bar in overgrip, cast to squat on low bar
    b) as in a) to stoop on low bar
    c) from stomach whip position, both hands on high bar in overgrip, beat swings
    d) stomach whip beat swing to squat on
    e) stomach whip beat swing to squat over to long hang swing
    f) stomach whip beat swing to stoop on
    g) stomach whip beat swing to straddle over to long hang swing
    h) stomach whip beat swing to stoop on
    i) stomach whip beat swing to stoop over to long hang swing

Basic Support Positions

Jump to front support—body straight, in overgrip   M   LB
Stride support—hands in overgrip   HR   LB

Rear support—hands in reverse grip	M	LB
1. "L" hold	HR	B
2. "V" hold	R	I
Free straddle hold	R	B

Basic Skills from Front Support Position

Cast to free front support and return to front support on low bar	M	LB
Cast, single leg flank to stride support		LB
Cast, single leg shoot through	HR	LB
1. squat through		
2. stoop through		
Cast, double leg shoot through	HR	B
1. squat through to rear support		
2. Squat through to "L" hold		
3. Stoop through to rear support		
4. Stoop through to "L" hold		
Cast to free straddle hold	R	B

Hip Circles

Kickover to back hip circle mount	M	LB
From low bar, kickover back hip circle to high bar	M	LB
Pullover to back hip circle mount	M	LB
Cast, back hip circle	M	LB
1. bent knees		
2. pike		
Front hip circle	M	LB
1. bent knees, hands on low bar in overgrip		
2. pike		
Hip circle combinations		
1. Front hip circle, cast, return to front support	HR	B
2. Front hip circle, cast, back hip circle	HR	B
3. Front hip circle, cast, back hip circle, underswing dismount	R	B
Free Hip Circle	R	HI

Stride Circles (Mill Circles)

Forward stride circle	HR	LB
Backward stride circle		B
Stride circle, catch high bar (Mill circle catch)	HR	B

Sole Circles

Back sole circle, straddle position	M	HB
1. Hands and feet swing in straddle position under low bar with hands in overgrip		
2. Jump from floor to straddle hang swing under the low bar		

3. From long hang on high bar, place feet on low bar in straddle position and alternately transfer hands to low bar in overgrip to sole circle dismount
4. From straddle stand on low bar holding high bar, alternately transfer hands to low bar in overgrip to sole circle dismount
5. Cast from front support on low bar to straddle sole circle dismount
6. From a stand on low bar, jump to straddle sole circle dismount from high bar
7. Cast from front support on high bar to straddle sole circle dismount facing away from low bar
8. Cast from front support on high bar to straddle sole circle dismount over low bar

Back sole circle, straddle position, ½ turn   M   HB

1. Cast from front support on low bar to straddle sole circle, ½ turn dismount
2. Jump or cast to high bar to straddle sole circle, ½ turn dismount
3. On low bar, cast to straddle sole circle, ½ turn with mixed grip to a stand on floor
4. Jump or cast to high bar to straddle sole circle, ½ turn with mixed grip to wrap in on low bar without releasing high bar
5. Cast to straddle sole circle, ½ turn on low bar, releasing both hands and regrasping low bar in overgrip to stand on floor
6. Jump or cast to high bar to straddle sole circle, ½ turn releasing both hands and regrasping high bar in overgrip to wrap in on low bar without releasing high bar

Back sole circle, stoop position   HR   LI
(can follow the same basic progressions as the straddle sole circles)
Back sole circle, stoop position, ½ turn   HR   LI
(can follow the same basic progressions as the straddle sole circle, ½ turns)

Front sole circle, straddle position   M   I

1. Hands and feet straddle swing under the low bar with hands in reverse grip
2. Cast to straddle position on low bar, hands in overgrip; jump to stand on floor
3. Cast to straddle position on low bar, hands in overgrip; switch hands to reverse grip and jump to stand on floor
4. From straddle stand on low bar, facing and grasping high bar, alternately transfer hands to

low bar in reverse grip and execute front straddle sole circle

5. Cast to straddle on low bar with overgrip; change hands to reverse grip, front sole circle
6. Cast to straddle on low bar with overgrip; reverse grip; front sole circle to glide or glide kip
7. From stand on low bar, jump to straddle position on high bar with overgrip; reverse grip to front sole circle
8. From front support on high bar, cast to straddle position; reverse grip to front sole circle

Front sole circle, stoop position	HR	I

(can follow the same basic progressions as the straddle front sole circles)

Seat Circles

Front seat circle	M	I

1. Pike compression hang under low bar with hands in reverse grip
2. "L" hold drill on low bar, reverse grip
3. Front seat circle

Back seat circle	M	I

1. Pike compression hang under low bar with hands in overgrip
2. "L" hold drill on low bar, overgrip
3. Basket swing
4. From a standing position (on spotter's knee or from spotting block) with body in a compressed pike position and hands in an overgrip, open to rear support on low bar while rotating grip
5. Back seat circle

Cast to free straddle support, back seat circle in straddle position (stalder)	HR	HI
Cast to straddle stand on low bar with hands in overgrip; change to reverse grip to front seat circle in straddle position	HR	HI

Kips and Kip Related Movements

Double leg stem rise	M	B
Single leg stem rise	M	B
Short kip—from low bar rear support to kip to front support on high bar	M	I
Drop kip from front support	HR	I
Glide kip	M	I
From front support, push away glide kip	HR	I
Glide kip, front hip circle, push away to glide kip	HR	I

Glide single leg overshoot to stride position on low bar	M	I
Glide double leg overshoot to rear support on low bar	M	I
Glide single leg overshoot, catch high bar	HR	I
Glide kip catch the high bar	M	I
Glide double leg overshoot, catch high bar	HR	I
From hang on high bar, drop glide kip catch the high bar	M	I
From rear support on low bar, single leg overshoot to stride position on high bar	HR	I
From rear support on low bar, double leg overshoot to rear support on high bar	HR	I
Long hang kip	M	I

    1.   from squat stand on low bar
    2.   from pike stand on low bar
    3.   from sitting position on low bar
    4.   from stomach whip, squat over low bar
    5.   from stomach whip, straddle over low bar
    6.   from stomach whip, stoop over low bar

Reverse kip	R	MD
Stomach whip, uprise to high bar	R	D
Straddle cut catch	HR	I

    1.   Basket swing—from "L" support on low bar, drop backward into pike compression swing and return to rear support
    2.   Basket to straddle cut dismount on low bar
    3.   Basket to straddle cut catch the low bar
    4.   Glide double leg overshoot, straddle cut catch
    5.   Short kip, straddle cut catch the high bar
    6.   Long hang kip, straddle cut catch the high bar

Wrapping Movements

Wraps initiated from the back of the high bar
(i.e., the side away from the low bar)

1. Long hang from high bar, push off low bar and wrap in	M	B

    a)   push off the low bar with hips by driving legs backwards while hips are still in contact with low bar
    b)   multiples of this swing wrap drill
    c)   when speed is sufficient, wrap the low bar by executing a back hip circle when hips contact the low bar

2. Cast to free front support on low bar and push away to stand on floor	M	B
3. Cast on high bar to coaches support	HR	I

Caution—arms should be kept straight. Bending arms allows the gymnast to drop straight

down increasing the possibility that hands may lose grip on high bar		
4. Cast wrap—cast from high bar to back hip circle on low bar to front support position	M	I
5. Cast wrap, eagle	M	I
6. Cast wrap, hecht	M	I

Wraps initiated from the front of the high bar
(i.e., the side near to the low bar)

1. From front support on low bar, one hand on high bar in overgrip and other hand on low bar in overgrip, beat off low bar to squat or stoop position on low bar	HR	LB
2. Stomach whip	M	LI
a) lying with hips on low bar, hands on high bar in overgrip, beat off bar and return		
b) Multiples of a)		
c) start from squatting position on low bar		
d) start from standing position on low bar		
e) start from cast from high bar		
3. Reverse wrap	R	I
a) from lying position on low bar, hands in overgrip on high bar, beat off low bar and return to back hip circle on low bar		
b) start from standing position on low bar		
c) start from front support on high and cast to reverse wrap		
4. Reverse wrap, hecht off low bar, passing under high bar	R	HI
5. Reverse wrap, eagle	R	A

Vaulting Mounts

Vault to back hip circle on low bar	R	B
Vault to front hip circle on low bar	R	B
Vault to squat over the low bar to long hang on high bar	R	I
Vault to straddle over the low bar to long hang on high bar	R	I
Vault to straddle position on low bar to sole circle catch high bar	R	HB
Vault to ½ turn, back straddle over the low bar to glide kip	R	I
From behind the high bar, vault to catch high bar in overgrip, straddle or stoop legs over low bar, immediate kip to high bar without touching low bar	R	HI
Vault to free hip circle on low bar to glide kip	R	A

Horizontal Bar: Areas of Concern

Physical and psychological readiness are essential for horizontal bar activities. If a gymnast cannot grasp the bar and touch his thumb to his fingers, he should not be taught skills involving rotation. Before working on the horizontal bar, the gymnast needs a highly developed kinesthetic awareness. He must understand the importance of normally rotating in the direction in which his thumbs point and of correct body mechanics in swings, dismounts, and recoveries in the event of falls. Above all, the gymnast must understand the difference between responsible courage and carefree daring.

Progression is extremely important and check-off charts are highly recommended for motivation. Beginners should start with basic skills. Most skills, even of the basic level, will require some minor hand spotting at the early stages. Elementary compulsory exercises, incorporating the basic skills, are advisable in order to stimulate adequate review of the fundamentals. These exercises will allow for the development of form and execution. Dismounts and recovery movements should be taught with each new skill.

An adjustable horizontal bar should be used for beginners. Many skills, whether basic or advanced, can first be learned on the chest-high adjustable bar before progressing to the jump-height competitive bar.

Safety precautions are essential because of the risks involved for both gymnasts and spotters. The instructor/coach should constantly check the condition of the apparatus, the adequacy of mats, and the availability of chalk. The supervising instructor/coach should make spotting rules appropriate to the type of gymnasts for whom he is responsible. In mature classes or teams, gymnasts may be permitted to work in groups of three on beginning skills, providing proper spotting has been mastered, thus allowing two spotters to give verbal and physical aid to the student on the bar. On advanced skills, the supervisor/coach is responsible for deciding when completion of a learning progression permits a gymnast to work safely without an overhead belt.

Safety Tips for Instructors and Coaches

1. Check apparatus before and throughout the activity. Make sure bar itself and supporting devices (floorplates, cables, turnbuckles, and attachments) are in safe condition, secured, and stable.
2. Use mats prescribed for competition plus additional mats for safe teaching of new or difficult skills, especially dismounts.
3. Check condition of gymnasts' hands and proper use of chalk.
4. Be sure a gymnast has the strength, physical and psychological preparation, and technique for each particular skill. Be sure he can grasp the bar and touch his thumb to his fingers before teaching rotational skills. Be sure he knows the importance of rotation in the direction his thumbs point, and how to change direction with a mixed grip swing. Be sure he understands the potential hazards to gymnast and spotter from the great amounts of centrifugal force and angular momentum in this activity.
5. Use a low bar for beginning skills.
6. Have enough spotters, properly positioned. Some type of spotting platform is recommended; a folded mat is effective and safe. Use safety belts when needed for safe spotting.

7. Train spotters thoroughly. Be sure they understand the desirability of spotting from below the bar, in order to avoid getting the spotter's arm between gymnast and bar. When the gymnast is in the air (free position), spotting should be done at or above the center of gravity or hips, in order to protect the gymnast's head and neck. A spotter should always know and make sure the gymnast knows which direction he will be going.

8. Train spotters to anticipate problems by understanding the mechanics of each skill. In rotational skills, the spotter should be able to anticipate a fall and the direction in which the gymnast is likely to go and thus take a saving position.

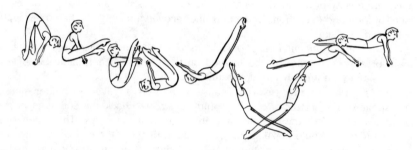

Horizontal Bar Progression (Men)

Training in basic skills, starting with a low bar, should precede the regular progression on the horizontal bar. A sequence of basic skills is given below, with recommended bar heights.

Many authorities advise a sequence of elementary compulsory exercises, incorporating the basic skills, before the regular progression is started. A scoring system can be used to measure the gymnast's mastery of fundamentals. A set of basic compulsory exercises used in many U.S. physical education classes is given below; for comparison, the Swiss Youth Program horizontal bar beginners class exercises also are shown. A scoring system is given with each set of exercises.

Elementary and Intermediate horizontal bar progressions follow the basic skills and exercises. The degree of difficulty, recommended bar height, and importance of each skill is noted. Those skills marked as "absolute musts" are essential to future skills of higher difficulty, and should never be bypassed. Those skills marked as "recommended" are important but not necessarily essential. Skills are grouped in three categories: Long Swings, Short Circles, Upstarts and Kips. These categories seem logical and useful to many instructors and coaches, but the experienced gymnastic supervisor may want to develop his own.

Basic Skills to Precede Elementary Horizonal Bar Skills

Key:

L.B.—Low Bar (chest height)
R.H.—Reach Height
J.H.—Jump Height (competitive)

Skills and Sequences	*Bar Height*
Front pull-over to front support	L.B.
Back inverted straight hang	L.B.
Back inverted German hang	R.B.
Pike hang	L.B.
Single leg upstart	L.H.
Front pullover from hang	R.H.
Back inverted pullover to rear support	L.B.
German hang release one hand to full turn regrasp	R.H.
L. hang to front pullover	R.H.
Cast to controlled under swing	J.H.
Cast to controlled swing to single leg upstart	J.H.
Underswing shoot dismount from stand on mat	L.B.
From front support, underswing to arch dismount forward.	R.B.
Underswing cast from support to intermediate swing	J.H.
From front support lower backward to front pullover	L.B.
Single crotch circle forward from support to support	L.B.
Single crotch circle backward from support (overhand)	L.B.
From crotch support, flank vault dismount ¼ turn	L.B.

Basic Horizontal Bar Compulsory Exercises
From a side stand frontwards:

1. Jump to hang with double overgrip and execute front pull-over to front support
2. Swing legs forward to underswing
3. On the forward swing, pass left leg between hands to single leg upstart
4. Change to undergrip and swing right leg over the bar with ¼ turn to the left and dismount to cross stand

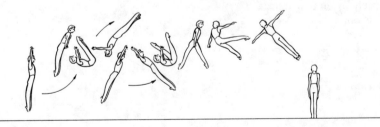

Skill	Value	Typical Faults	Deductions
1.	3.0	Visible sign of strain	.3 to .5
		Legs not straight	.2 to .4
2.	2.0	Swing not smooth	.2 to .5
		Extra swing	.5 each time
3.	3.0	Leg bent when passing between hands	.2 to .4
		Failure to reach sitting position on	
		first attempt	.2 to .5
4.	2.0	Left leg bent on swing over bar	.1 to .3
		Poor position of body on dismount	.2 to .3
	10.0		

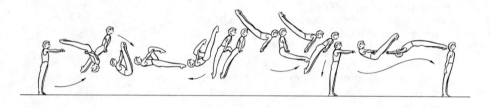

SWISS YOUTH PROGRAM
HORIZONTAL BAR (CHEST HIGH)
BEGINNERS CLASS

	Value
Stand chest high over grip, Front pullover to support.	2.0
Fall back slowly and hook L or R knee.	2.5
Single leg upstart, bring forw. leg sideward and back to front support.	2.5
Cast to backward hip circle to bounce on mat, followed immediately by an underswing shoot dismount.	3.0
	10.0

Elementary and Intermediate Horizontal Bar Skills

Key: *Degree of Difficulty*   *Importance*
     E   Elementary   R   Recommended
     LI   Low Intermediate   M   Absolute Must
     MI   Medium Intermediate
     HI   High Intermediate

Skills and Sequences	Degree of Difficulty	Importance	Bar Height
LONG SWINGS			
Simple forw. and backw. swings (overgrip)	E	M	J.H.
Simple forw. and backw. swings with ½ turns	E	R	J.H.
Backw. uprise from hang and underswing	E	R	J.H.
Upward swing to front support	E	M	J.H.
½ forward giant to front support	E	M	J.H.
Underswing from support to back uprise	E	M	J.H.
Underswing ½ turn mixed grip to kip	E	M	J.H.
Underswing ½ turn change grip, kip	E	R	J.H.
Back uprise from underswing mixed grip	E	R	J.H.
Underswing ½ turn mixed grip, ½ giant	LI	R	J.H.
From support, cast back, reach under with ½ turn to back uprise	LI	R	J.H.
Back uprise, squat through to rear support	LI	R	J.H.
Back seat circle from rear support	LI	M	L.B.
Back uprise squat through to back seat circle	LI	R	J.H.
Back uprise to flank catch rear support	LI	R	J.H.
From support one forw. giant (undergrip)	MI	M	J.H.
From support one back giant (overgrip)	MI	M	J.H.
Cast out forw. from rear support to L swing, full turn at back (undergrip)	MI	R	J.H.
Forw. circle in rear support (undergrip)	MI	M	L.B.
Forw. circle rear support shoot forw. dismount	MI	R	L.B.
Back uprise from high underswing to straddle rear support (overgrip)	MI	R	J.H.
Same as above with straddle seat circle backward	MI	R	J.H.
Single leg double rear from back uprise swing to straddle seat fall back	MI	R	J.H.
Flank vault catch to rear support	MI	R	J.H.
Flank vault catch mixed grip	HI	M	J.H.
Back uprise, flank catch in L position swing forward ½ turn to kip	HI	R	J.H.
Reach under mixed grip, flank catch	HI	R	J.H.
Free back hip circle to above	HI	R	J.H.
¾ forward giant, change over grip to reach under ½ turn mixed grip, flank catch	HI	R	J.H.
High underswing with release and full turn catch at back of swing	HI	R	J.H.

SHORT CIRCLES

Forward hip circle	E	M	L.B.
Backward hip circle	E	M	L.B.
Drop kip to forward roll	E	R	L.B.
From front support squat legs through to jump	E	R	L.B.
Underswing to straddle under bar to rear support in straddle position	LI	R	R.H.
Same as above continue to seat circle	LI	R	R.H.
Underswing with mixed grip, squat under bar, shoot legs backward to inward ½ turn to regular grip	LI	R	J.H.
From rear support, undergrip circle forw.	LI	M	L.B.
From rear support, same to shoot dismount	LI	R	L.B.
Front support, squat through and same as above	LI	R	L.B.
Rear support to back seat circle overgrip	LI	R	L.B.
Rear straddle support, same as above	LI	R	L.B.
Rear support, cast backw. to German, land on mat (½ German)	LI	M	L.B.
From rear support int. swing backw. to flank regrasp regular hang	MI	R	R.H.
Same as above to straddle catch	MI	M	R.H.
Back uprise to free hip circle handstand	HI	M	J.H.

UPSTARTS AND KIPS

Regular forw. upstart overgrip	E	M	R.H.
Regular forw. upstart undergrip	E	M	R.H.
Drop kip from support to support	E	M	L.H.
Front support underswing mixed grip ½ turn kip	E	R	R.H.
Same as above except with under grip kip	E	R	R.H.
Mixed grip underswing, ½ turn to overhand kip	E	R	R.H.
Swing double hop change at front swing from over to underhand grip and kip	LI	R	R.H.
From support cast back and same as above	MI	R	R.H.
With overgrip kip and cast to handstand	MI	M	R.H.
With undergrip kip and cast to handstand	MI	M	R.H.
Kip with overhand to double hop to undergrip	MI	R	R.H.
Strong kip, ½ hop change to regular giant backward	HI	R	J.H.

10

The Trampoline and Gymnastics Programs

The trampoline has become integrated with many physical education and recreation programs, and is often used as a training aid for sports including gymnastics. Use of the trampoline in gymnastics programs is accepted by the United States Gymnastics Safety Association, provided such use complies with the general provisions of this manual and the specific provisions of this chapter. Safety provisions for the minitramp are similar to those for the trampoline, but a special comment on the minitramp appears at the end of this chapter.

With the popularity of the trampoline has come the desire to learn and experiment. Unfortunately many unrealistic ideas, poorly reasoned concepts, and dangerous practices have arisen from a shortage of sound instruction. Trampolining is no more hazardous than many other physical activities, but it offers such a challenge that a trampoline user may become carried away with his success—or seeming success. Because of this potential over-confidence, supervision (as defined in Chapters 2 and 12) is crucial at all times.

Location and Staff Availability

Before integrating the trampoline with a gymnastics program, an instructor or coach should make sure there is a safe place for the apparatus to be used, according to the guidelines in Chapter 2. He or she also may wish to consult the Standard Consumer Safety Specification for Components, Assembly, and Use of a Trampoline, published by the American Society for Testing and Materials (ASTM; see Selected Bibliography). In addition to checking the features of the physical environment, as discussed in Chapter 2, the instructor or coach should be guided by the following recommendations:

1. Overhead clearance above a trampoline should be adequate for safe use according to the skills being taught or practiced.
2. A level surface should be provided with no obstructions beneath the trampoline.
3. A well-lighted area should be provided for trampoline activities.
4. Facilities should be available to secure trampolines against unauthorized or unsupervised use. If the apparatus cannot be kept in a locked room or storage area, it should be folded and secured with a chain and padlock.

Advance planning to insure adequate supervision is another prerequisite for safe use of trampolines. Before a trampoline is acquired, the instructor or coach should

---

Illustrations in this chapter are from Jeff T. Hennessy, *Trampolining*, copyright © 1968 William C. Brown Co., Dubuque, Iowa 52001. Used by permission.

be sure that enough trained staff members are available to provide appropriate supervision, according to the guidelines in Chapter 2 and this chapter.

Selection, Assembly, Care, and Maintenance of Trampolines

Trampolines should be selected in accordance with the guidelines in Chapter 3. Also helpful is the ASTM Standard Consumer Safety Specification, noted previously.

The manufacturer's instructions should be studied by the instructor or coach so that he or she is familiar with the trampoline's mode of assembly, use limitations, and care and maintenance requirements.

If a trampoline must be transported, a person familiar with the apparatus should be present to supervise the move. Care should be taken that the unit is secure before it is moved, and that enough persons are present to handle its weight. If a trampoline is to be folded or unfolded, care should be taken to follow procedures recommended by the manufacturer and to make sure the persons performing the task have adequate strength and skill (see this chapter's Beginning Lesson Plan). Improper moving, folding, or unfolding of a trampoline can result in damage to the apparatus and/or injury to the persons involved.

Before every class or session in which a trampoline is used it should be inspected by a qualified person, according to the manufacturer's recommendations and the following checklist:

1. Sagging bed
2. Holes or worn places in the bed
3. Deteriorated stitching in the bed
4. Ruptured springs
5. Bends, breaks, or missing parts in the frame
6. Protrusions of the frame or suspension system
7. Missing or improperly attached frame pads

Worn, defective, or missing parts should be replaced or repaired in accordance with manufacturer's specifications. In addition to proper frame pads securely attached to the trampoline, floor mats should be appropriately placed. See Chapter 4 for proper selection, installation, care, and maintenance of floor mats. Generally, Basic Mats should be placed on the floor around a trampoline, although these may be omitted at ends equipped with large spotting decks.

Spotting

An adequate number of spotters—with sufficient strength, alertness, and training— should be in position before each activity in which a trampoline is used. See Chapter 5 and the remaining sections of this chapter for suggestions about the selection and training of spotters, especially the utilization of students for spotting. Note particularly that responsibility for safety is always the teacher's, not the student spotter's—and that spotting is a multifaceted skill which must be learned.

Four basic procedures are used in trampoline spotting:

1. Floor level spotting
2. Spotting with an overhead mounted belt

3. Bed level hand spotting
4. Bed level hand belt spotting

Floor level spotting has the objectives of preventing a trampoline user from coming into contact with the frame or falling to the floor. The number of floor level spotters—as well as their strength, alertness, and skill—should be adequate to protect the trampoline user.

Spotting with an overhead mounted belt is often appropriate for teaching new skills (see Chapter 5). The pulleys should be centered on both sides of the trampoline, far enough apart to avoid entanglement of the trampolinist's arms in the supporting ropes. With the safety belt around the waist of the trampolinist, the spotter pulls down on the ropes while the trampolinist springs up, and feeds out the ropes as the trampolinist drops to a landing on the trampoline bed. The spotter must keep time with the up and down rhythms and at the same time maintain maximum control over the actions of the trampolinist.

Bed level hand spotting is done in three ways. A first method requires a spotter to stand on the bed with both feet, grasping the trampolinist in an appropriate manner, "giving" with the up action and gently depressing the bed as the trampolinist lands. A second method requires the spotter's feet to leave the bed and return with the trampolinist's. A third method requires a spotter to keep one foot on the frame pad and one on the bed, lifting the foot on the bed in rhythm with the trampolinist's movements and stepping onto the bed when assistance is needed. Bed level hand belt spotting follows the principles described in Chapter 5, with the two spotters standing on the frame pads on each side of the trampolinist. *Note:* All methods of bed level spotting require great skill, so those desiring to master these methods should consult the trampolining books listed in the Selected Bibliography, by the author of this chapter and others, and should obtain adequate training from qualified instructors.

Programs of Instruction

A physical educator must distinguish trampolining activities included in school and college physical education programs, those used for training team gymnasts, and those offered by organizations and specialized schools and camps.

Following are criteria for using trampolines in physical education classes. These are similar to those adopted by the American Alliance for Health, Physical Education, and Recreation, in Position Statements cited in the Selected Bibliography.

1. That the program be elective.
2. That the program be supervised by trained personnel.
3. That spotters be in position when the trampoline is in use.
4. That somersaults *not* be allowed. (An exception may be made for advanced students with demonstrated proficiency when belt spotting is available; see AAHPER Position Statement.)
5. That the trampoline be kept locked when not in use.
6. That regular inspection of the trampoline be conducted.
7. That policies for emergency care be preplanned.
8. That accident records be kept for the trampoline, as well as other gymnastic apparatus.

Note that somersaulting skills are specifically excluded from regular physical education classes. Also, special care should be exercised with any skill involving rotation around the lateral axis where the body may become inverted. In general, the physical education instructor has a particular responsibility in selecting trampolining skills appropriate to the physical and psychological preparedness of the students.

A gymnastic coach has a similar responsibility except that he or she typically can assume a higher level of preparation among team members than among physical education students. Even among varsity athletes, freedom from belt spotting in skills involving the somersault should be permitted only at high levels of proficiency (see AAHPER Position Statements). The coach's task is likely to be in the direction of restraining over-confidence—and of confining trampolining activities to those which enhance gymnastic skills.

The instructor in charge of a specialized program for trampolinists is not bound by criteria such as those of the AAHPER nor by the limits of standard gymnastic events. His plan for a trampolining program, therefore, must draw upon his entire experience and the experience of others such as the authors listed under Selected Bibliography.

Areas of Concern

Lax supervision, unsound instruction, inadequate spotting, and, above all, an *indifferent attitude* are the main problems in supervising trampolining activities. Instructors or coaches seldom are indifferent because they do not care about the trampoline user but rather because they do not *know the risks* involved. Trampolines can propel the user to unaccustomed heights and into unfamiliar body positions, so teacher and student must overcome a psychological barrier of indifference in approaching this apparatus. True familiarity with the trampoline will breed respect for its potential.

Temptation to depart from experience-tested progressions is another concern. The would-be trampolinist should understand that he or she is seeking mastery of a skill requiring *progressive steps* from basic bounces and body positions to recognized activities of a more advanced nature; that departures from these steps involves risk of injury.

Safety Tips for Instructors and Coaches

1. Inspect the trampoline before each class or session when it is to be used, in order to be sure it is in a safe position and fully operational.
2. Assure yourself that all users of the trampoline are in suitable physical and psychological condition—not fatigued, "silly," or under the influence of alcohol or drugs.
3. Be sure appropriate supervision has been provided before a trampoline is unlocked: specific supervision for beginners learning basic skills or for more advanced trampolinists learning new skills; general supervision for all participants and bystanders in the gymnasium.
4. Make sure adequate spotters and spotting equipment are in place.
5. Warn all participants of the risks involved in departures from lesson plans or in "horse play."

Beginning Lesson Plan (minimum duration of 5 to 6 weeks)

Because only one person at a time is permitted to use a trampoline, a class should be organized for the most effective use of available time. Division of a class into groups of ten is recommended in order to allow one trampolinist and nine floor level spotters per trampoline at any time. (Smaller groups may be desirable, provided the number of spotters is adequate.) A system of rotation should be organized so that each student, as he or she completes a turn, dismounts at the place of mounting. This procedure enables the teacher to keep track of students' turns and to be sure of adequate floor level spotting.

All students should be instructed in floor level spotting and advised of the importance of their role as spotters. Every group should understand that all members are *active participants at all times,* not only in spotting but also in observing and appreciating the skill being performed on the trampoline.

During the first class session, students should be given the following:

1. Short history of trampolining
2. Names of the parts of the trampoline and explanation of their functions
3. Necessity of taking care of the trampoline and keeping it in good working order
4. Demonstration of how to fold and unfold the trampoline (accompanied by warning against undertaking these operations without teacher's permission, based on an assessment of students' strength and skill)
5. Experience in folding and unfolding the trampoline (omitted for smaller children)
6. Basic safety rules and the reasons for their enforcement
7. Demonstration of how to mount, how to do the basic bounce and the check bounce, and how to dismount (with warning against jumping off the trampoline in any circumstances)
8. Experience in following these procedures

Trampoline Progression (Men and Women)

New skills should be demonstrated before students attempt them, and students should assume the basic positions involved for purposes of orientation. All twisting skills should be in the same direction preferred by the student. The presentation of new skills should be kept to a minimum height so that control can be mastered. Basic skills should be developed to the point where every student feels confident and can perform with poise.

A recommended progression follows. The number of skills which can be mastered in five to six weeks by a given class will depend on the students' level of ability. Mastery of a part of the listed activities is preferable to halfhearted coverage of the whole list.

Basic Skills

1. Basic bounce
2. Check bounce
3. Change of direction (twisting around the longitudinal axis)
4. Tuck jump
5. Straddle jump

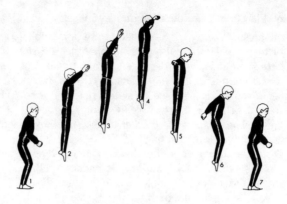

Basic bounce and check bounce

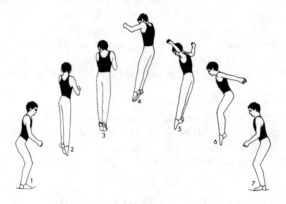

Change of direction (twisting around the longitudinal axis)

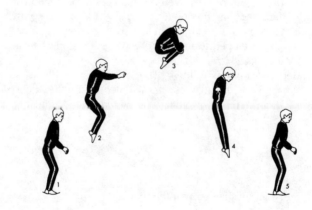

Tuck jump

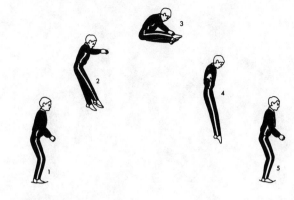

Straddle jump

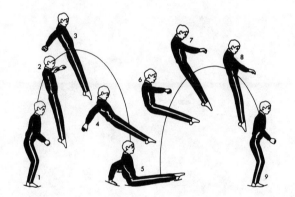

Seat drop

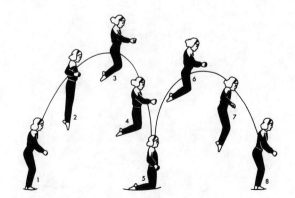

Knee drop

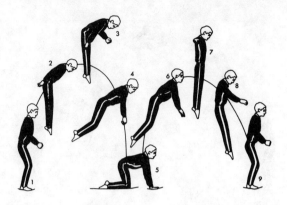

Hands and knees drop

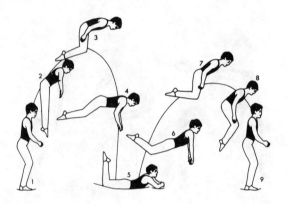

Front or stomach drop

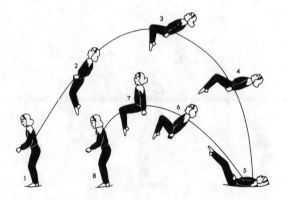

Back drop

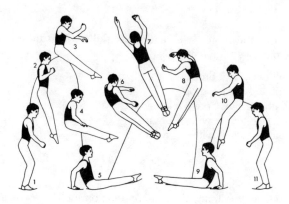

Swivel hips

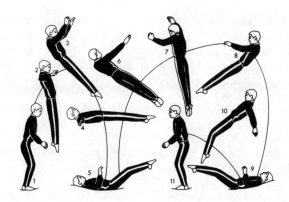

Cradle

6. Seat drop
7. Knee drop
8. Hands and knees drop
9. Front or stomach drop (This first should be performed from a hands and knees drop.)
10. Back drop
11. Swivel hips (seat drop, 1/2 twist to seat drop)
12. Cradle (back drop, 1/2 somersault with 1/2 twist to back drop)
13. Swingtime—a procedure of doing one skill right after another without a free bounce between skills
14. Add-one—a game where each student must do what the previous student did, then add a new skill (This game should be confined to the level of skills learned during class.)

Additional Skills

Upon completion of the basic skills, additional skills within the same range of difficulty can be presented, such as

1. Seat drop, full twist, seat drop
2. Back drop, full twist, back drop
3. Front drop with 1/2 twist to a back landing
4. Back drop bounce to feet with 1/2 twist
5. Seat drop bounce to feet with 1/2 twist

Minitramps

A minitramp is similar to a trampoline in construction, but is designed for single-contact activities followed by landings on mats. Safe use of the minitramp, therefore, requires precautions similar to those for the trampoline combined with those recommended for vaulting.

Location and Staff Availability. The location of a minitramp should follow the general guidelines in Chapter 2 and those for a trampoline. But there are three differences. For a minitramp, adequate horizontal and vertical clearance is necessary to avoid collisions, as it is in vaulting; and space must be available for appropriate landing mats, as described in Chapter 4. Finally, because of the way a minitramp is used, care should be taken to place it on a nonskid surface. Adequate staff must be available to supervise the use of the minitramp and to prevent its misuse.

Equipment. Selection, assembly, care, and maintenance of minitramps should follow the guidelines of this chapter and of Chapter 3. Inspection before each activity using the apparatus is essential. Landing mats, as described in Chapter 4 for vaulting activities, are of crucial importance. Supervisors are responsible for insuring minitramps against unauthorized use.

Spotting. Adequate floor level spotting—as outlined in this chapter for the trampoline—should be provided for the minitramp. In addition, hand and belt spotting should be provided for dismounts in the landing area, as described in the Vaulting section of Chapter 9.

Programs of Instruction. The AAHPER position statement on trampolines (see Selected Bibliography) contains the following paragraph on the minitramp: "As recommended for trampoline safety, the minitramp should constitute an elective activity requiring competent instruction and supervision, spotters trained for that function, emphasis on the danger of somersaults and dive-rolls, security against unsupervised use, proper erection and maintenance of the apparatus, a plan for emergency care should an accident occur, and documentation of participation and of any accidents which occur."

The United States Gymnastics Safety Association adds these recommendations for the use of the minitramps in physical education classes or in the training of gymnastics team members: first, no skills should be allowed which involve contact with more than one minitramp in the same exercise; second, in regular physical education classes no skills should be allowed which terminate on any part of the body other than the feet; third, skills involving somersaults or dive-rolls should be restricted to advanced gymnasts and skilled spotters; fourth, multiple somersaults should not be allowed in regular physical education classes, and single somersaults should be permitted only with the utmost discretion.

Use of the minitramp in recreation programs—under the sponsorship of organizations or specialized schools and camps—should follow practices found safe and effective by the supervisory staffs and by the authors cited in the Selected Bibliography. There is no substitute for informed experience to assure the safest possible conditions in any activity.

11

Medical Responsibility in the Gymnasium

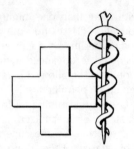

Prevention of mishaps is the first responsibility of the gymnastic instructor or coach, as this manual has emphasized in every chapter. Since some accidents are bound to happen in a sport requiring skill and exertion, preventive measures must be accompanied by preparation for medical emergencies. Statistics show that accidents are the chief cause of death among persons between one and 38 years old, according to the American National Red Cross, but community studies show that medical care education can significantly improve the likelihood of victims' recovery. The ABCs of medical care preparation are:

A. Always have Medical Information Forms for each gymnast (see suggested form at end of chapter), in order to know of any physical or psychological handicaps he or she may have—including chronic ailments such as diabetes, epilepsy, heart disease, allergies, or asthma—as well as the name of his or her physician and relatives to be notified in emergencies.

B. Be ready to summon help from the most appropriate source: a physician, a certified athletic trainer, an ambulance service, a person trained in the American National Red Cross Advanced First Aid and Emergency Care program, or a person trained in the Red Cross or American Heart Association resuscitation program. (Leaders of high-risk or high-exposure activities should themselves receive emergency medical care training, according to a recommendation of the National Academy of Sciences/National Research Council.) A telephone should be available to every gymnastic instructor or coach, and posted near it should be numbers for

Ambulance (or Emergency Operations Center)
Team or School Physician
Athletic Trainer
Fire Department (or Emergency Operations Center)
Police Department (or Emergency Operations Center)

C. Carry an adequate amount of emergency care equipment and supplies. This should be stored in a safe and accessible place such as the gymnasium office; should be plainly marked; and should be inspected periodically to assure its cleanliness and usability. A minimal first aid kit should contain:

"Band-Aid"-type bandages
4x4 gauze dressings
adhesive tape
"Kling"-type bandages
multi-trauma dressings
air-splint set

triangular bandages
Mild soap (not detergent)
water basin (water source should be available)
blankets
sheets
pillows
sand bags

Emergencies Resulting from Gymnastic Mishaps

Organizers of athletic contests or meets are responsible for providing adequate professional medical help for any athlete—or spectator—who may need it. During training or practice the instructor or coach is responsible for care of the injured until professional help is available. If a physician or emergency care specialist is not available at all times on a moment's notice, the instructor or coach—or a regular assistant or staff member—should take Red Cross or equivalent training (see B above). Such training should be updated as required through refresher courses. Following are a few first aid suggestions for the most likely gymnastic-related medical emergencies.

Shock. Every serious injury to the human body causes a condition called *shock* resulting in depression of bodily functions. The best way to prevent shock is to treat every injured person as if he is suffering shock. A victim should be placed on his back with his legs elevated, unless this position aggravates an injury to the head, chest, or leg. Since chills occur with shock, normal body temperature should be maintained by the use of a sheet or blanket. Care should be taken to make sure no airway obstruction is present, and nothing to eat or drink should be given to the injured athlete.

Soft-Tissue Injuries. Perhaps the most common injury in any athletic situation involves damage to the soft tissue of the body. In gymnastics a common example is an avulsion injury to the hand of an individual performing on the horizontal bar. This may result in a large portion of the skin being torn from the surface of the hand. For any type of soft tissue injury, medical follow-up care will be necessary, and in an injury like the one described here may involve surgical procedures. For a soft-tissue injury, the coach's responsibility should merely be to control external hemorrhage and prevent aggravation of the injury. Direct pressure and a pressure bandage almost always suffice to control blood loss in this type of situation. Once bleeding is controlled and the athlete can be removed from the gymnasium, he should be immediately referred to further medical care. Extensive cleansing or debridement of the wound is not warranted in the gymnasium since this will be part of follow-up care. When cleansing appears to be indicated—that is, if the wound does not involve tissues deeper than the skin—mild soap and water is usually the best initial treatment.

Orthopedic Injuries. The next most common injury received in any athletic activity involves damage to the bones and joints. Often these injuries involve the soft-tissue surrounding the joint, increasing the level of pain experienced by the athlete. If the injury involves a joint or a possible fracture, the injured part should be immobilized (splinted) and the athlete transported to a medical care facility capable of performing x-rays and providing physician support. In certain minor injuries, the supervising instructor or coach may be able to immobilize the injured area with any one of a variety of splinting devices. If the athlete is to be transported to the hospital by ambulance, it is best to leave him/her in the position discovered and allow the qualified emergency medical technician to immobilize the injury before transportation. Further injury can result from improper splinting technique, and the individuals qualified for providing ambulance service have experience in immobilization technique.

Cardiopulmonary Arrest and Airway Obstruction. The cessation of respiratory or cardiac activity in the gymnast is an unlikely occurrence. It is conceivable that some younger athletes could be affected by upper airway obstruction from foreign matter such as a piece of candy held in the mouth while performing an activity. If a gymnast's airway becomes obstructed and he/she is still trying to expel the obstructing object by coughing, the victim should be encouraged to do so. If the victim has ceased to breathe or has become unconscious, the rescuer should perform the airway clearing techniques prescribed by the American Heart Association's Committee on Emergency Coronary Care. Techniques to relieve airway obstruction require special training and practice. These procedures should not be attempted unless specific training has been received through the American National Red Cross or the American Heart Association.

It is possible that someone of any age could receive traumatic injury or could suffer from an illness that may result in the cessation of spontaneous respiratory and cardiac activity. In the event that this occurs, the coach may be the only one in the area who can initiate the immediate steps necessary to save the life of the athlete. Head injury alone can result in respiratory arrest, and the simple technique of cardiopulmonary resuscitation can effectively stabilize the victim's condition until further medical care can be obtained. If the technique is not performed, the victim of a head injury may die. Given the high speed performance of some gymnastic events and the potential contact with apparatus, such a head injury is within the realm of possibility. Once again, before such techniques are attempted, the individual performing the resuscitation should have attended a training program sponsored by either the American National Red Cross or the American Heart Association.

Central Nervous System Trauma. The most alarming injury that may occur to an athlete involves injury to any part of the central nervous system from the cerebral cortex and skull to the lower spine. Perhaps the most common injury involves damage to the cervical spine area. If such an injury occurs, immediate immobilization is mandatory. Without adequate immobilization of a cervical spine or neck injury, temporary and/or permanent paralysis may result. There are a number of methods for immobilization of individuals with neck and back injuries. The simplest temporary measure for neck injuries is to place sandbags beside the head and neck on *both sides*. More sophisticated techniques require many hours of practice to perfect. If the supervisor or coach of a gymnastic activity suspects the possibility of cervical spine injury, the victim should not be moved under any condition, and qualified medical help should be summoned immediately. This qualified medical help may include the team physician, the athletic trainer, and the ambulance service responsible for your immediate area. The athletic team physician and trainer can provide on-site evaluation and management. Unless the ambulance service is called immediately, the athlete's transportation and subsequent medical care may be significantly delayed.

Emergencies Resulting from Chronic Conditions

The instructor or coach is responsible for the well-being of athletes under his supervision, whether or not their ailments result from gymnastic activity, no matter if he has full Consent, Waiver, and Release Forms on file.

The instructor or coach must have every athlete's significant medical history at hand in case of an emergency resulting from, or complicated by, a chronic condition. For instance: If a gymnast should suffer insulin shock, an asthmatic spasm, an epileptic seizure, or a heart attack, the instructor or coach must report the underlying condition (if any) to emergency medical personnel in the event the gymnast's regular physician or parents cannot be reached. If a tetanus shot seems called for, the instructor or coach must know whether the athlete is allergic to such an innoculation. At a camp the instructor or coach must know of gymnasts' plant or insect bite allergies.

The Medical Information Form below is designed to prepare the instructor or coach for any emergency resulting from a chronic condition. Information should be taken from every gymnast's latest medical examination report, and missing items should be reported to proper authority. Forms should be accessible to assistants or staff members who may be temporarily in charge of gymnastic programs. Medical records should be preserved after a student's departure from a course or team, in the event of a legal controversy (see p. 115).

Supervisory Responsibility

The possibility of injury in gymnastics demands that every supervisor (1) be aware of potential medical emergencies, (2) be prepared to meet them. If there is any chance of delay in obtaining medical help, the supervisor—or regular staff assistant—should be capable of providing initial care. Certification by an accredited organization such as the Red Cross attests that emergency care training meets current standards. The supervisor is responsible for making sure that such certification is kept up-to-date through refresher training.

MEDICAL INFORMATION FORM FOR GYMNASTS

Participant _____ _____ _____
                        (name)   (age)   (sex)

Physical Handicaps   *Psychological Handicaps*
(Specify missing or injured bodily   (Specify problem areas such as anxieties,
parts, weaknesses, etc.)   fears, hyperactivity, hypersensitivity.)

bones and joints _____   _____

muscles _____   _____

organs _____   _____

weight problem _____   _____

Chronic Ailments   *Allergies*
asthma, or other respiratory problems   insect bites _____

_____   tetanus shots _____

circulatory or heart problems   other, if significant _____

_____   _____

diabetes or hypoglycemia _____   *Blood type* _____

epilepsy _____   *Current Medication (if any)*

hemophilia, or other bleeding problems

_____   _____

Physician Who Conducted Examination

_____ _____   _____
        (name)   (phone no.)   (date of latest examination)

Preferred Personal or Family Physician(s)   *Health Insurance (if any)*

_____ _____   _____
        (name)   (phone no.)   (name of insuror)

_____ _____   _____
        (name)   (phone no.)   (policy no.)

Parent(s), Guardian(s), or Other Relatives   *Employer (if any)*

_____ _____   _____
        (name)   (phone no.)   (name)

_____ _____   _____
        (name)   (phone no.)   (phone no.)

_____ _____
        (name)   (phone no.)

116

12

Legal Responsibility in the Gymnasium

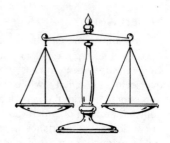

Lawsuits seem to be a way of life, and anything is fair game—including you as a gymnastics coach or instructor. You should not allow a fear of being sued prevent you from having a good gymnastics program. There is really no point in being scared that you will be sued—you cannot protect yourself 100%. Be realistic about lawsuits and about safety practices: be aware of aspects of a program's operation which may give rise to a lawsuit. Set forth in this chapter is a series of guidelines which will help minimize the likelihood of suits being filed, and if suits are filed, these guidelines will serve you well as a defense. The principles are synthesized from the law as evidenced in state statutes and over 1,000 cases which have been reviewed in the field of athletics, physical education, and recreation.[1] It should be pointed out that the law varies from state to state, jurisdiction to jurisdiction, and in case law, precedence can be changed with the next case before the court. The guidelines are basic, however, and should give you a good foundation for conducting your program and for your defense, if necessary.

The overriding question is—*With what standard of care must you perform?* It is frequently heard that one must be "a reasonable and prudent person," but that is not enough—you must be a *reasonable and prudent professional.* An individual must have the competence required for the role he is performing. If you present yourself as a physical educator and are teaching gymnastics, then you are claiming you know the proper procedures for gymnastics. Further, if you are not a physical educator but are coaching gymnastics, you are held to know not only the techniques of gymnastics but also relevant aspects of the student gymnast's psychological and physiological development. It is irrelevant as to whether you actually do know . . . the court will hold that you *must perform* as if you are fully qualified to do that which you have undertaken; that is, you must perform in a professional manner.

What is professional conduct? In general, a key aspect is that the individual be up-to-date on the "best practices" of the profession. This requires a particular concern for gymnastics and a continuing education relating to the desirable practices of coaching and teaching gymnastics. This manual provides an excellent beginning on desirable safety practices; however, one must keep professionally up-to-date as new safety equipment is developed or new procedures recommended. The guidelines presented in this chapter are principles of professional conduct and the specifics of gymnastics must be applied. The principles of professional conduct are divided into three categories: supervision, conduct of the activity; and environmental conditions—equipment, facilities, and areas.

Supervision

Supervision of participants in activity is one of the critical elements giving rise to lawsuits. Two types of supervision—general and specific—should be distinguished. General supervision means that an individual must be within the activity area overseeing the activity, while specific supervision means being at the specific location of activity with the participants. The nature of the supervisory actions is dependent on the type of supervision required. The distinction between the two types is of considerable importance if you have a large physical education class, an athletic squad practice, or persons participating in a recreational program—obviously the instructor or coach cannot be with each individual all the time. When *must* he or she be directly with the person engaging in activity providing specific supervision and when is general supervision adequate?

General Supervision There are three considerations for general supervision. First, the supervisor (instructor, coach) must be *immediately accessible* to anyone who needs him; he must never leave the premises, for to do so opens wide the door for lawsuits. If injury occurs, some competent person must be secured either to take care of the injured or supervise the participants. Further, the supervisor must be able to oversee the entire program systematically; that is, rotate to all parts of the activity area. For example, in one case an 18-year-old youth was in a gymnastic class for his physical education requirement.[2] The class met twice a week for 50 minutes, but it was usual for the students to remain after class to work on individual skills and thus perfect certain stunts. This practice was encouraged by the instructor. One day after class the young man was using the large trampoline attempting to perform a double-forward somersault when he lost his balance and fell off the trampoline onto the floor, landing on his head and shoulders, sustaining serious permanent injury. There was one student spotting. The instructor at the time was 30–40 feet away assisting another student on the horizontal bar. There were five students in the gym. The rule in class required four spotters for performance on the trampoline, but the number after class varied with the situation. The young man was a skilled performer and participated in the Youth Circus. The court held that there was no negligence on the part of the instructor. Thus supervision at each piece of apparatus being used was not required. However, there seems to be some case precedent that there must be a *plan* of supervision. In one instance, the physical education faculty had been given the responsibility of general supervision of the gymnasium area.[3] The teacher on duty was sitting at his desk with his back to the window, when two boys became engaged in "slap boxing" and one was seriously injured. The court held that there was no plan for supervising and that certainly just being on the premises was not supervision.

Second, in general supervision one must be alert to conditions that may be dangerous to participants. A professional should not only be able to identify dangerous conditions but also anticipate such conditions and establish accident-prevention procedures. These conditions include defective premises or apparatus, lack of protective devices, mats, or safety equipment, and participants going beyond their capability—these conditions will be described in subsequent sections and recommended practices specific to gymnastics are presented in the foregoing chapters of this manual. Dangerous conditions also include rowdyism and poor discipline. One of the largest awards in legal history for personal injury to a single individual for negligence ($4,025,000) went to a fifth-grade boy who was permanently disabled in a summer recreation program sponsored by a city recreation and park department on a school playground.[4] He was hit on the side of the head by a larger boy during a scuffle over which child was to take a turn at bat in an organized ball game. Bleeding inside the skull resulted in a blood clot forming and exerting pressure on the brain stem, causing muteness and paralysis from the neck down. At the time of the injury a male supervisor was responsible for the boys on the playing field and a female supervisor was giving instruction in arts and crafts inside. The male supervisor had left the field, presumably to assist the female supervisor, but there was conflicting testimony as to the length and nature of his absence. The male supervisor, however, knew that fights among the boys were frequent and that part of his job was to stop or prevent them. Probably, if appropriate general supervision had been given, the injury would not have occurred. A person cannot be an insurer of safety, however, and the court tries to be reasonable. In a basketball game, one player without provocation struck an opposition player in the face with his fist causing injuries of a serious nature.[5] It was alleged that the player who hit the other player was not properly supervised and controlled—not so, the court held.

One question which frequently arises is how much force a person can use in disciplining. In a physical education class, a 14-year-old, 4-foot 9-inch tall, 101-pound boy did not participate as instructed and the teacher (34 years old, 5 feet 8 inches tall, 230 pounds) ordered him to the sidelines.[6] The ball rolled toward the boy standing on the sidelines and the teacher ordered the boy back when he entered the court to retrieve the ball. The boy then again tried to rejoin his shooting line on the court and the teacher physically disciplined him by escorting the boy from the court, and when they reached the sidelines the boy tried to strike the teacher, upon which the teacher grasped the boy's arms to restrain him. The boy alleged that the teacher chased him around the court, caught him, lifted him from the floor with a "bear hug," shook him against nearby bleachers, and dropped him to the floor, fracturing his arm. The court held that a teacher has the right of restraint, but that in this situation he went beyond the restraint necessary and used excessive physical force. Undue force can bring a charge of assault and battery. Sometimes an instructor tries to justify force and discipline based on the doctrine of *in loco parentis,* that the action is to safeguard the child as a parent would. However, under this doctrine one is a guardian of general welfare only and may discipline a child only to protect him from severe self-injury.

Rowdiness control extends to spectators and to extracurricular activities; thus appropriate arrangements must be made for crowd control (usually working with local police or campus patrol) and for adequate supervision of club activities.[7] The area of disciplining rowdy participants and crowds is one which might well be included more often in professional conferences and workshops.

The third consideration for general supervision is first aid and emergency care. The nature of the relationship between instructor/coach and participant requires that the instructor/coach be knowledgeable in first aid. In an early case it was held that had the supervisor been found (general supervisor must be immediately accessible), she would have known first aid and would have stopped arterial bleeding which took the life of a small girl.[8] The immediacy and nature of the first aid administered is frequently in issue. For example, a young man died of profound heat exhaustion with shock to an advanced degree when improper procedures were followed.[9] The high school football team began practice at midafternoon and near the end of the session, during wind sprints, the young man staggered and became faint. The coach removed him from the workout and sent him to the school bus (the field was a distance from the building with showers). About 20 minutes later when they arrived at the school, the young man was assisted into the school, placed on a blanket on the floor, his clothing removed, and immediately given a shower with water at room temperature, then covered with a blanket, and was offered a drink of salt water, but was unable to drink. A physician arrived about 3 hours after the initial symptoms of distress. The court held that the coaches delayed medical aid too long after symptoms appeared and in addition applied ill-chosen first aid. A landmark case highlights the frequent concern for proper moving of an injured player—the injured person could move the extremities, but after improper moving was paralyzed.[10]

Not only knowledge of first aid but also continued refresher work stressing the most current and best practices—and the ability to recall immediately the appropriate first aid required by the symptoms—are of utmost importance in preventing injury, and provide a good defense when injury does occur. It must be pointed out that to hold a certificate for first aid and emergency care is *no protection* regarding negligence—it is the *actual act* that is evaluated in court. A certificate is only evidence to an employing administrator that an individual has been exposed to certain first aid knowledge and practice and supposedly has a certain level of competence in rendering first aid. However, a generalized first aid certificate is inadequate—*the knowledge of first aid must extend to those injuries most likely to occur in gymnastics,* and greater emphasis in training must be placed on first aid for such injuries. (See Chapter 10, Medical Responsibility for recommended practices.)

Specific Supervision Two considerations in regard to specific supervision are parallel: when introducing an activity you must stay with the participant until he is familiar enough with the activity to evaluate his own capacity to do the activity and to understand and adhere to safety practices and procedures which have been established, and the parallel, when an activity is going on under your general supervision and you note any failure to adhere to rules and regulations or you see some change in the condition of a participant, such as overfatigue or apparent lack of appreciation of dangers, then you must change from general to specific supervision. Specific supervision involves appreciation of the activity in terms of one's capacity to do the activity, and understanding and adhering to safety practices and procedures.

The appreciation of risk is essential both for the safety of an individual and for the use of the defense of assumption of risk in a lawsuit. It has often been said, especially in sports, that the participant assumes the risk of the sport, but cases in the 1970s have put a new emphasis on the responsibility of the supervisor of the activity. *A participant does not assume any risks he is not aware of and does not appreciate!* This places the burden on the coach/instructor for appropriately *communicating risks involved and being certain the participant understands.* Knowledge of risk is not sufficient. Some have referred to this informing and subsequent participation as "advise and consent," but there is much more to this advising and consenting than appears on the surface. It is important that it be noted that knowledge of a risk is insufficient; that is it is not sufficient to merely inform or warn of risks in an activity. There must be an understanding *and appreciation of* that risk. This appreciation of risk works both ways; that is, the inexperienced participant requires greater effort on the part of the coach/instructor to communicate the risks; on the other hand, if a performer is young but experienced, he is held to assume those risks of which he is knowledgeable and should appreciate. For example, in the case cited under general supervision, the young man on the giant trampoline was an experienced and skilled performer. The court held that a proficient performer must exercise the same judgment and discretion in care for his own safety as a person of more advanced years when on a trampoline. With such experience, the instructor was justified in providing only general supervision. Similarly, the court held in a softball case that the injured was an "intelligent young man" who had played without protective eyeglasses for several years and had had proper warnings of danger not only of the protective equipment but also regarding standing behind the batting cage screen, which tended to "give" when a ball was hit into it; thus the injured person assumed the risks in participation.[11]

The risks one assumes are those normal to the activity itself. An individual has the right to expect that the equipment is not defective, that the safety devices will be adequate, and that the instructions given are correct, and when this is not true, these become negligent acts and a person does *not* assume any risks due to negligence; a person does not give "license" to anyone to be negligent at his expense. Too often the signing of a "permission slip" by parents for a child to participate or the signing of a "waiver" by an adult is misunderstood—all such signatures mean is that they will assume the *normal* risks of the activity, *they do not give permission for a coach/instructor to be negligent.* Permission slips are useful public relations strategy, for they both deter suits and inform as to what a person will be doing, and for such purpose it is recommended that they be used. (Coincidentally, a spectator also assumes the risks of the game, such as a fly ball into the stands at a baseball game, but does not assume risks due to defective safety devices, such as a backstop which does not stop a ball.)

A key to assumption of risk is the appreciation of the risk in relation to the condition or capacity of the individual for performing the activity. The instructor/coach must be a communicator par excellence to help the participant evaluate his own capacities in regard to the difficulty and requirements of the activity. For the instructor/coach to do this requires considerable professional skill (see next section, Conduct of the Activity). There must be an understanding of the activity itself and what it requires, as well as of the individual's physical condition and psychological mood. The coach should be able to identify changes in the condition of a participant, both physically and psychologically, which would endanger the safety of the individual. Specific supervision must be given when such symptoms are noted until there is assurance that it is safe for the individual to continue, or else the individual must be removed from the activity. An understanding of the psychology of sport, as well as of the anatomy, kinesiology, and physiology of human development, as related to gymnastic performance, is essential.

The second concern for specific supervision relates to safety practices and procedures. Appropriate safety practices and procedures must be established, and these must be particular to the activity being undertaken, rather than generalized safety practices and procedures; that is, there may be some general regulations in the gymnastics area and then safety procedures specific to certain apparatus and activity thereon. Each sport has its own requirements, and a person instructing or coaching must be familiar with them. Other chapters in this manual give suggestions regarding such regulations and practices.

When a new activity is introduced there must be specific supervision, but as the performer becomes more proficient, general supervision is adequate. If, however, under general supervision some change in the physical or emotional condition that might endanger the individual is noted, or if a violation of safety practices and procedures is observed, then the instructor/coach must immediately give specific supervision until the situation is once again safe.

Lack of Supervision as Proximate Cause While lack of supervision is a most frequent allegation in negligence cases, such lack of supervision must indeed be the cause of the injury. We are not and cannot be insurers of safety, and supervision will not prevent all injuries! For example, during the Christmas holiday six boys persuaded the gymnasium custodian to let them use the basketball court. Two went for a loose ball, hitting their heads, and one was seriously injured.[12] It was alleged that there was a lack of supervision—there may not have been supervision, but supervision certainly could not have prevented the injury. Similarly, three teen-age boys were racing in a pool (appropriately racing) when a 15-year-old boy dove into their paths, and one boy was seriously injured.[13] Certainly with no previous notice of horseplay by such person or at the pool in general this action could not have been anticipated, and lack of supervision was not the proximate cause.

Conduct of the Activity

The courts have not held any activities except boxing inherently hazardous. This is not to say that some activities, and some gymnastic apparatus and routines, do not involve more risks and thus require more of the participant both physically and mentally, and therefore more care of the instructor/coach, but it does say that the risks which give rise to lawsuits are based in negligence of people, not hazards of activity. Therefore, this section on conduct of activity is of special importance. Negligence occurs when one owes a duty to protect, in this specific situation, a person engaged in gymnastics, from the unreasonable risk which might foreseeably harm him, and such duty is not performed adequately. There are three aspects of particular concern relating to the conduct of the activity: adequacy of instruction and progression; maturity and condition of participant; and warning of danger or dangerous conditions.

Adequacy of Instruction and Progression If you give instructions to a participant and he is injured, you are liable—if your instruction was inadequate or did not communicate the degree of risk. This requires an understanding of the activity in terms of appropriate technique and progression. (See especially Chapter 9, Progression in Teaching Skills for recommended practices.) In one of the best known early cases, a high school sophomore girl was required to enroll in a beginning tumbling class over her objections and to perform 10 of 18 different types of stunts, including the "roll over two," to get a passing grade.[14] The injured testified that she was not given instruction directly by the instructor on the stunt "roll over two," but that she was shown how to do the exercise by advanced students. She also said she had fallen many times in doing the exercise and had a bad knee, which the instructor knew about. The girl sustained a skull fracture when she performed the exercise incorrectly, bending her arms so that her hands and head hit the floor at the same time. In a questionable decision, the injured did recover when the court held the exercise not suitable. Inadequate instruction and lack of supervision were involved in another case where the injured and a classmate collided on a mat while doing a somersault.[15] In a 1973 case a 17-year-old boy was attempting to do a forward roll gymnastic exercise on a set of still rings when he slipped and fell to a floor mat.[16] He was still classed as a beginner although this was his third year, and it was the seventh week of nine. The stunt was considered easy. The safety rules required orientation, spotters, and "ask for help." On the day of the accident, he had been asked about his spotters, but didn't get one for himself, and said he "forgot." The court held that the instructor gave adequate supervision and instruction. In another rings case, an 11-year-old fifth-grade girl was injured while performing on the rings in gymnastic class under direction of a certified physical education teacher.[17] She stood up in the rings and in jumping out, fell backward, landing on her back. She had done this dismount on other occasions and had also seen others do it, and there had been no objection from the teacher. The teacher denied that she had ever seen the girls do it, although admitting it was a dangerous practice. At the time of the accident, the teacher's back was turned. The state syllabus said regarding apparatus that the class should be entirely in the view of the teacher.

Maturity and Condition of the Participant It is here that professional competence—both knowledge and judgment—is essential. One must not only know how to teach a skill technique but also understand the human being biologically and psychologically and the relationship of physical activity thereto. To relate to maturity and condition, the progression and sequencing of activities is extremely important. The coach/instructor must sufficiently know the capacities and capabilities of his students so that appropriate groupings and activities may be used in relation to characteristics of the participant. Such considerations include understanding the stage of development of the individual from a maturing point of view, as well as the physical condition and psychological state of the individual. (See especially Chapter 8, Physical Preparedness for recommended practices.) Where there are required activities, an adopted syllabus of activities, progression by grade level, either district or state, is desirable.

Several cases involve the physical condition of the participants. In one situation a 17-year-old high school junior was injured when performing the exercise "jumping the buck."[18] She alleged that she had weak wrists and had told the teacher, but was forced to do the exercise anyway. When her wrists gave way she pitched forward, causing injury. An exercise known as "knee walk" being done by a high school girl was involved in another case.[19] She noticed a dull ache and tiredness in her left knee, and as she performed the next exercise, "inch worm," she felt a sharp pain on her left side and collapsed sideways upon the floor. The pain seemed to localize in the left knee. The court found no negligence in supervision and held that an accident is not necessarily due to negligence.

Regarding the age of the participant and the appropriateness of apparatus, there is a case in which a first-grade pupil fell while hanging from a 6-foot-high horizontal bar.[20] The court held it was appropriate that the child should be on this particular bar. The opposite result was reached when a 6-year-old, although told not to use it, was playing on a 7-foot-high horizontal ladder 30 feet long. He became exhausted, fell, and broke his arm.[21]

Also for special consideration under this particular topic should be the increasing participation by girls in sports, including gymnastics. There are many myths regarding girls and participation, both psychologically and physiologically. There is no reason to refer to an activity as "for girls." The same principles hold—the individual, whether a boy or a girl, must have the strength, endurance, physical condition, psychological set, and experience required to do the activity. The progression is the same.

Warning of Danger or Dangerous Conditions As previously noted, activities in themselves are not dangerous—but the way in which they are conducted may be. There is an obligation to provide a safe environment and to warn of dangerous conditions. Dangerous conditions for different activities may vary. A coach/instructor working with gymnastics must know what dangerous conditions there might be specifically for gymnastics. This particularly involves the use of safety devices, such as protective mats and spotters. (See especially Chapter 4 on mats, Chapter 5 on spotting, and Chapter 6 on personal equipment.) Several previously mentioned cases referred to spotting. In another case it was alleged that the teacher was negligent in not having placed mats under the chinning bar; however, the accident occurred in the preclass warmup period to a performer who had done the routine many times before and was of sufficient skill and knowledge to put his own mats down if he wanted them. It was stated that in this situation with a drop of only 6 inches from the chinning bar, mats were not essential for safety but were there to cushion the drop.[22]

In addition to giving instructions regarding spotting and protective devices, which is the best way to ascertain whether or not the participants are comprehending what to do and the importance, warnings may also be given as printed literature (signs, pictures, posted printed regulations), which provides an ever-present reminder of the importance of safety procedures. While such warnings are very useful and should be given, the instructor still has a responsibility to check that desirable practices are being followed and that the participants appreciate the importance of using safety equipment and aids. Integral to this aspect of warning of danger is the establishment of procedures for safety rules and regulations. (See Chapter 7 on the use of visual aids.)

Environmental Conditions

Whereas the preceding section dealt with dangerous conditions and a safe environment as related to the activity, this section continues in its concern for safe environmental conditions, but focuses on the physical facilities and area. (See also Chapters 2 and 3 on gymnasium facilities and apparatus.)

Equipment A participant in the assumption of risk of an activity does *not* assume the risk of defective equipment. Proper maintenance and care of equipment is of utmost importance. Where defective equipment is known, it is the instructor/ coach's responsibility not to use it. Defective equipment includes improper installation of equipment and inadequate maintenance.

The court held that a balance beam which had just been varnished and placed on a newly oiled floor constituted a continuing dangerous condition when an 8-year-old boy was injured in a fall.[23] Appropriate care must also be taken when installing new equipment. For example, the installing company had left a 250-pound horizontal ladder lying on the ground over a holiday. The principal had told the children to stay away until the equipment was completely installed; however, an 8-year-old and other children attempted to lift the ladder and it fell on the 8-year-old, injuring him. The court held that the ladder was not inherently dangerous and no recovery was awarded.[24]

One important point should also be made regarding "locking" equipment. Usually, particularly on playgrounds and general gymnasium equipment, to lock an area or facility is really no protection against use of defective equipment. If a person gets into a locked area and is injured on the equipment out of use due to defect, the courts usually find for the injured person.

Facilities There are several considerations relating to facilities. The first of these relates to the physical condition of the gymnastics area, such as the floor: if there are loose boards which might give rise to injury, inappropriately padded walls, or lack of safety glass—beware. Also, the condition of the shower can be important: an improperly rinsed disinfectant may make the floor slippery; the floor in places where it is usually wet may lack nonslip surfacing; lockers may be poorly anchored or in need of repairs.

One legal concept that is especially important as related to both equipment and facilities is that of notice or knowledge of dangerous conditions. There are two types of notice, actual and "constructive." With actual notice, the dangerous condition has been called to the attention of the responsible party: one has actual knowledge about the situation. Constructive notice, on the other hand, means that one should have known about the situation had he appropriately inspected or been aware of what was taking place. A person is liable for both! Once one has notice, then there is a duty to take action to remedy the dangerous condition. Sometimes a dangerous condition has arisen suddenly, but there has been a regular inspection or observation of conditions; appropriate time for notice may be allowed before liability attaches. The key issue is how diligent the person was in seeking out dangerous conditions, and then with what expediency the remedial action was taken.

Another aspect of facilities usually taken care of by the administration, but about which a coach/instructor should be aware, is the condition of the bleachers. The "owner" of the facility is liable for the condition of the bleachers, and in nearly all lawsuits brought when bleachers have collapsed the injured parties have recovered awards.

Defenses

The best defense, of course, is that there was *no negligence,* that in fact the act was performed according to the appropriate professional standard. It is to that end that the foregoing discussion has been given. The second primary defense, also previously discussed, is the assumption of risk by the participant; however, it has been indicated that there must be knowledge and understanding of the risk involved in the activity and that the risk assumed is only for those normal risks involved in the activity and does not include risks of inadequate supervision or instruction or defective equipment or other negligence.

The doctrine of governmental immunity, which a few jurisdictions still have related to schools, is not truly a defense. Rather, it means that the corporate entity (school) is not subject to being sued. This doctrine, however, has been abolished or modified in many (state) jurisdictions and should not be relied upon. To abolish the doctrine in any given state requires only one case or act of the legislature. Furthermore—and often misunderstood—the immunity is only for the corporate entity and does not protect the individual or coach.

Some technical defenses can be used, primarily that the statute of limitations has run. In this case, an individual injured while a child has until the statute of limitations (usually two years) has run after his reaching majority. Thus it is very important that a record of accidents be kept until past that time. Because of crowded court dockets in some jurisdictions, records there should be preserved three to five years beyond statutory limits. Several states have passed "notice of claim" laws, that is, within a certain number of days (ranging from 30 to 120 days, depending on jurisdiction) the injured person must give "notice" that he intends to sue. Usually there are strict procedural requirements for such notice. Several states have held these laws unconstitutional as in conflict with statute of limitations, while about the same number of states have held them constitutional.

What about insurance? Of course, insurance is not a defense. It is a way of protecting against undue financial loss in case negligence should be found and a large award is made. It also is used to handle small nuisance claims, which are frequently "paid off" in an out-of-court settlement. Where insurance is carried, the legal staff of the company handles claims and court actions. An employee (instructor, coach) should be sure to check whether his employer's insurance covers the employees; not all do! However, in a few states there is what is known as a "save harmless" or indemnification law which requires the employer to cover its employees.

Often "waiver" forms and parental permissions are considered a defense—but, as previously indicated, these are good public relations devices that do little when negligence is involved. These basically indicate that one acknowledges that they rightfully assume the risks normal to the activity, but they do not give license to those conducting activity to be negligent or for the activity to be conducted on dangerous facilities or equipment.

"Ten Commandments"

In summary, to minimize the likelihood of being sued, and to assist in a sound defense if you are sued, the following guidelines are recommended:

1. A procedure for accident emergencies, including a complete accident form, should be established.
2. A plan for supervision should be established.
3. In-service education with emphasis on (a) developmental needs and capabili-

ties of participants, (b) first aid and emergency procedures, and (c) safety procedures for activities is a must.

4. Safety rules, regulations, and procedures should be established *and enforced.*
5. *Accident insurance* should be carried; this will minimize many of the liability suits if the injured person does not have to make a large financial outlay.
6. There should be regular inspections of facilities, areas, and equipment, and an A-1 program of maintenance, especially preventive maintenance.
7. Programs should be based on a progression of activities in accord with human development, skill, and experience, and sufficiency of leadership and appropriate equipment/facilities/area.
8. Competent personnel only should be used.
9. Good public relations programs should be established, including parental permissions.
10. Consult your local attorney and insurance carrier.

Philosophically, we should recognize that:

We are apt to be sued; it is the attitude of the times and there are more people participating and hence more possibility of injuries; don't let a suit "throw you" emotionally.

We cannot prevent suits by eliminating activities from our programs; people seek risk which requires physical and mental courage; the task is to help them participate in the safest possible manner.

We are not insurers of safety, but are accountable to conduct a program and keep areas and facilities in a condition that does not promote unreasonable risk.

People sue when something irritates them—so watch your public relations! Take care of the injured and cover as much of the expense as possible; establish procedures for prompt care and notification of next of kin.

NOTES

1. van der Smissen, Betty. *Legal Liability of Cities and Schools for Injuries in Recreation and Parks* (including Physical Education and Athletics). W.C. Anderson Company, Legal Publishers, Cincinnati, 1968 with 1975 supplement.
2. *Chapman* v. *State,* 6 Wash App 316, 492 P 2d 607 (1972).
3. *Dailey* v. *Los Angeles Unified School District,* 84 Cal Rptr 325, vac. 87 Cal Rptr 376, 470 P 2d 360 (1970).
4. *Niles* v. *San Rafael,* 116 Cal Rptr 733 (1974).
5. *Fustin* v. *Board of Educ.,* 101 Ill App 2d 113, 242 NE 2d 308 (1968).
6. *Frank* v. *Orleans Parish School Bd.,* 195 S 2d 451 (1967 La App).
7. *Aaser* v. *Charlotte,* 265 NC 494, 144 SE 2d 610 (1965).
8. *Bellman* v. *San Francisco High School District,* 11 Cal 2d 576, 81 P 2d 894 (1938).
9. *Mogabgab* v. *Orleans Parish School Bd.,* 239 S 2d 456 (La 1970).
10. *Welch* v. *Dunsmuir Joint Union High School District,* 326 P 2d 633 (Cal Dist Ct App 195).
11. *Hanna* v. *State,* 46 Misc 2d 9, 258 NYS 2d 694 (1965).
12. *Albers* v. *Indp. School Dist.,* 94 Idaho 342, 487 P 2d 936 (1971).
13. *Benoit* v. *Hartford Accident and Indemnity Co.,* 169 S. 2d 925 (La 1964).

14. *Supra* n. 8.
15. *Clark* v. *Board of Educ.*, 304 NY 488, 109 NE 2d 73 (1952).
16. *Lueck* v. *Janesville,* 204 NW 2d 6 (Wis 1973).
17. *Tardiff* v. *Shoreline School Dist.*, 68 Wash 2d 164, 411 P 2d 889 (1966).
18. *Cherney* v. *Board of Educ.*, 31 App Div 2d 764, 297 NYS 2d 688 (1969).
19. *Ostrowski* v. *Board of Educ.*, 31 App Div 2d 571, 294 NYS 2d 871 (1968).
20. *Cordaro* v. *Union Free School Dist.*, 11 App Div 2d 804, 220 NYS 2d 656, aff'd 11 NY 2d 1038, 183 NE 2d 912 (1962).
21. *Howard* v. *Tacoma School Dist.*, 102 Wash 442, 173 Pac 335 (1918).
22. *Fein* v. *Board of Educ.*, 305 NY 611, 111 NE (2d) 732 (1953).
23. *Bush* v. *Norwalk,* 122 Conn 426, 189 Atl 608 (1937).
24. *Goldstein* v. *Board of Educ.*, Hempstead, 24 App Div (2d) 1015, 266 NYS (2d) 1 (1965), aff'd 18 NY (2d) 991, 278 NYS (2d) 224, 224 NE (2d) 729 (1966).

13

Teacher Certification Program of the USGSA

The United States Gymnastics Safety Association is a nonprofit organization with headquarters in Washington, D.C. It is sponsored by gymnasts, clubs, schools, camps, and industry for the PROMOTION OF SAFETY THROUGHOUT THE ENTIRE GYMNASTIC COMMUNITY.

All fees, dues, and instructional requirements for all classes of members and for certification tests are determined by the Board of Directors.

National Certifiers nominated by Board of Directors and inducted as USGSA Certifiers will initiate certification tests and have the duty to choose experts in their state areas to assist in conducting and administering certification tests for Gymnastic Safety Teaching Certification.

Applicants for certification must be paid-up members of USGSA or must pay an administrative fee equal to the first year's dues. Before admission to a certification course applicants must pay the course registration fee.

A recertification program is being developed by the USGSA Board in collaboration with other experts on gymnastic education. Recertification is essential for gymnastic safety, just as it is for emergency medical care, because of scientific and technological advances as well as changes in the social environment. Both certification and recertification are for two-year periods.

The Safety Teaching Certifications by the USGSA are supplements to a college degree in physical education similar to the Red Cross Swimming and Water Safety Courses. A college degree in physical education with courses in gymnastics does not necessarily meet the standards of Safety Teaching as promoted by the USGSA. An additional one-day course specifically designed for safety education is recommended by the Board of Directors.

Neither does a Safety Teaching Certification by the USGSA indicate complete prerequisites for successful teaching. The major objective of this certification program is to *reconfirm* an allegiance to a positive, working safety concept.

As the USGSA grows and incorporates more and more people, safety in gymnastics should be commonplace. The certification procedure will serve in developing *more awareness* of the responsibility carried by those who teach and coach.

Thus the certification programs are designed for those who are to teach aspiring gymnasts, especially young people, in order to make them more knowledgeable and qualified in both established and new areas.

Most of the men and women interested in teaching gymnastics will seek certification and recertification. The coaches and teachers who have national or international credentials will be asked to act as lecturers and to administer examinations to others seeking to be certified.

Certification is not an immunity to lawsuits, but it is an honest attempt at specialized training to help carry out the duty to discipline, supervise, and instruct with reasonable foresight and care. (Approved by USGSA Board of Directors)

Requirements for Gymnastic Safety Teaching Certification

Age

Minimum 18 years

Prerequisite

Knowledge of first aid.
Knowledge of some of the basics of gymnastics.
Attended clinics.
Assisted in class, camp, or school.

Competency

Must have a minimum of 100 contact hrs. as gymnast, assistant or student teacher, or coach.

Instructor Experience

Participated, coached, or judged gymnastics or participated in gym school or gym camp.

Course Text

THE GYMNASTICS SAFETY MANUAL of the USGSA

Evaluation Requirements

Must have registered, attended lectures, and passed written examination administered at a certification course.

APPROVED BY USGSA BOARD OF DIRECTORS

Note: Contact the USGSA Washington, D.C. office for scheduled Safety Certification Programs and a list of approved National Certifiers.

Recommended Minimum Time Table and Outline for Safety Certification Courses

Time	Topic	Personnel
9:00- 9:30	Registration, Fees, Forms, Time Table, Manuals	Certification Coordinators Secretarial Assistant
9:30- 9:45	Introductions of Staff and Guests, Course Agenda	Host Director State Chairman
9:45- 10:00	Philosophy— Ethics and Purpose	Master Clinician
10:15- 11:00	Legal Liability, Safety and the Law, Acts of Negligence, Standard First Aid Review, Emergency Procedures, Questions and Answers	Master Clinician Panel of Experts
12:00- 2:00	Lunch, Rest, Study of Manual, Handouts	
2:00- 2:30	Equipment and Facilities, Mats, Maintenance, Areas for Each Activity, ASTM, Gymnasium Inspections, etc.	Master Clinician Assistants
2:30- 3:15	Progression Learning Mens/Womens Events, Spotting Techniques, Demonstrations	Master Clinician Demonstrators Assistants
3:15- 3:30	Question and Answers about Test and Other Problems	Master Clinician Director of Certification
3:30- 4:30	Written Certification Test	Secretarial Assistants Clinicians
	Dismissal—test results to be mailed	

The USGSA will issue specific instruction to all National Certifiers prior to programs.

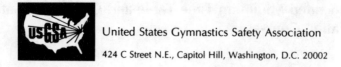

United States Gymnastics Safety Association

424 C Street N.E., Capitol Hill, Washington, D.C. 20002

Sample Form—Actual Form at Course Registration

REGISTRATION FORM FOR CERTIFICATION COURSE
(Please Print Information)

Name _____Sex_____Age_____

Address _____

_____Phone (___)_____

Business/School Address_____

_____Phone (___)_____

Affiliation_____Position/Title_____

Part I GYMNASTIC BACKGROUND

Circle number of years as a gymnast; coach; judge:

Gymnast 1 2 3 4 5 6 7 8 9 10 11 12 13 14 or more years____
Coach   1 2 3 4 5 6 7 8 9 10 11 12 13 14 or more years____
Judge   1 2 3 4 5 6 7 8 9 10 11 12 13 14 or more years____

List your accomplishments, position, or involvement in the following roles:

Gymnast_____

Coach _____

Judge _____

Administrator, Writer, Contributor, Student_____

_____

Graduate of _____High School_____College _____Others

Part II How many meets, clinics, congresses have you attended in recent years?
(Circle number.) 2 4 6 8 10 12 14 16 18 20 more ____.

How many instructional or learning programs have you been involved in during the
last five years (courses, workshops, seminars, summer camps)?

1 2 3 4 5 6 7 8 9 10 11 12 13 14 15, or more____

132

Part III Will you be taking an active part in gymnastics this season?

No_____ Yes_____

If yes, in what position and where?_____

_____

Have you ever taken a Certification Test by the USGSA before? Yes_____ No_____

If yes, were you certified? _____

Part IV As accurately as possible rank your capabilities on a scale of 1 to 10 in the following categories (1-novice, 3-beginner, 5-intermediate, 7-advanced, 9,10-expert, professional):

Teaching women's gymnastics	1	2	3	4	5	6	7	8	9	10
Teaching men's gymnastics	1	2	3	4	5	6	7	8	9	10
Spotting women	1	2	3	4	5	6	7	8	9	10
Spotting men	1	2	3	4	5	6	7	8	9	10
Understanding new trends and techniques	1	2	3	4	5	6	7	8	9	10
Keeping up with world and national gymnastic news	1	2	3	4	5	6	7	8	9	10
Understanding of progression	1	2	3	4	5	6	7	8	9	10
Knowledge of first aid	1	2	3	4	5	6	7	8	9	10
Care and an appreciation of the responsibilities of a teacher/coach	1	2	3	4	5	6	7	8	9	10

Any other comments? _____

_____

_____

_____

Applicant's Signature

(Do not fill spaces below.)

Signature of the Certifier_____date_____

Results of the Certification Test: Score _____ Passed _____ Failed _____

(This application must be forwarded to the USGSA office for recording and filing.)

Critical Review
of Books on Gymnastics

It has been more than ten years since the last comprehensive reviews of the gymnastic literature were reported.[1] The present review is an update of the one in the first edition of this Manual, eliminating a number of volumes which have gone out of print and utilizing a thorough reading of all gymnastic books published in the Seventies. The appended bibliography is a carefully selected list of publications currently available. The list has been broadened by the inclusion of a number of foreign language texts thought to be of value to the English reader, most of which are highly illustrated. Any gymnastic library holding a majority of the books listed here could be rated "excellent."

At present, many American gymnastic classics have gone out of print, and we have seen the subject matter of our field embraced by a number of publishers new to gymnastics. All of the books appearing in the reviews cited as well as those listed in the current editions of *Books in Print, Paperback Books in Print,* and *British Books in Print* have been screened to develop the list recommended here. Several publishers have also supplied outlines for books to be published in the near future.

The review and bibliography include some popular books written especially for the gymnastic enthusiast and the layman since 1976. There are quite a few such popular books in print and they are readily available in most large bookstores. Those selected are thought to be the best. For example, Straus's *Gymnastic Guide,* a collection of readings about gymnastics, would be a good reference for the sport reporter and other laymen who have had to rely on Menke's *Encyclopedia of Sports* for their insight. Tatlow's *The World of Gymnastics* is also in the category of a general reference with a collection of photographs by top gymnastic photographers such as Albrecht Gaebele, Alan Burrows, and our own Glenn Sundby. There has also been a growing list of books for youngsters relating life stories of their favorite stars. Cathy Rigby, Olga Korbut, and Nadia Comenici have all had one or more such volumes devoted to their life and times. The appearance of these books is a sure sign of the rate of growth of gymnastics in the United States, which has accelerated in the Seventies and has been reinforced by acquisition of gold medals by Kurt Thomas (a book about Thomas is in preparation) and Marcia Frederick, the first such honors to be carried off by Americans.

Although these books represent significant trends in the sport of gymnastics in the United States, they will not be treated further in this review. The purpose here is to suggest a number of books that would represent a small but excellent selection for the teacher/coach.

---

1. Frederick, A.B., "The Golden Library of Gymnastics," *The Modern Gymnast,* May/June, 1965, pp. 24–25; Frederick, A.B., "The Complete Book in Gymnastics," *The Modern Gymnast,* Feb., 1968, pp. 20–21; Berkowski, Robert, *Independent Gymnastic Survey,* Mimeo., n.d.

A Brief Critique

Although the decades preceding 1980 have produced precious few gymnastic texts that might be deemed theoretical in nature, there are definite signs that the English-speaking clinician may finally have some technically competent works to select from in the Eighties. *The Advanced Study of Gymnastics,* edited by John Salmela, is an example of the type of material found only in foreign-language publications up to the time of its first printing in 1976. One of the contributors to this compendium, Gerald George, published *Biomechanics of Women's Gymnastics* in 1979. George has been almost single-handedly responsible for the Biomechanics Task Force of the United States Gymnastic Federation (USGF) and he has sought out researchers in the gymnastic field to make presentations at the annual Congress of the USGF. Both Salmela and George are consulting editors to a new *Technical Supplement* to the *International Gymnast* which has a world-wide circulation.

Most books that are in print present a clinical approach to gymnastics, that is, they are written as a direct result of personal experience. Few supply the reader with any pertinent documentation and existing research, some of which includes practical applications for the coach. Research is still generally ignored. The same absence of documentation is also apparent in articles submitted to coaching journals which treat a variety of gymnastic topics.

Illustrations are still sufficiently weak to reemphasize the efficiency of film-drawn sequences that clearly demonstrate points made by the author. Cooper's *Feminine Gymnastics* includes sequences from film exclusively. The use of photography is still amateurish in most texts. The best example of illustrative photography in a gymnastic text is that of Kaneko's *Olympic Gymnastics.* The author has taken great pain to provide the reader with the best examples possible and the photographic excellence more than makes up for the unusual translation of terms from the Japanese, some of which would be unrecognizable without illustration. The popular Schmid/Drury text (*Gymnastics for Women*) now has an elongated female figure which improves the quality of their work.

The gymnastic text continues to be event-oriented rather than movement-oriented. This is a convenient method of distributing the author's material, but it does little to elucidate certain genealogical relationships among movements in a single family or class. West's *The Gymnast's Manual,* now out-of-print, was the only text in English to deviate from this event-oriented organization.

The Gymnastic Library

The books noted in the categories that follow are thought to be the best available for the gymnastic library. All of the books noted are in print, and details about obtaining them are found in the appended bibliography.

Children

Gymnastics is one of the most popular activities for children in the elementary school. There are several suggestions for materials at this level. O'Quinn's *Gymnastics for Elementary School Children* is an excellent resource with many ideas for multiple use equipment. Some of the pre-school instructional excellence of the German program has become available in an English translation of Liselott Diem's two-volume series entitled *Children Learn Physical Skills.* Her books contain many ideas for the pre-schooler and could be used in the development of a successful mother-child program in many of our gymnastic clubs, community-school programs, and in continuing education.

There are two other excellent sources of material for elementary school gymnastics. In one category are the publications such as those of the British Amateur Gymnastic Association (95 High St., Slough, Berkshire SL1 1DH, England) and the Canadian Gymnastic Federation (333 River Rd., Vanier City K1L 8B9, Ontario, Canada). Both organizations produce age-group materials which are superior to any obtainable in the United States. The second source of materials is associated with a creative program commonly known as "Movement Education." Plays Inc. (8 Arlington St., Boston, Mass., 02116) is the best source of materials for educational gymnastics. They are the U.S. distributor for the works of Laban and the very practical book by Mauldon and Layson entitled *Teaching Gymnastics*. Most of the better texts in this field are from British publishers.

Conditioning

The only book exclusively devoted to training methods for the gymnast is Spackman's *Conditioning for Gymnastics*. Spackman has also developed a personalized training program for athletes in a variety of sports including gymnastics. This program utilizes a pamphlet-like diary as a motivator for the athlete to concentrate upon those weaknesses that are discovered during testing.

Part Five of the Salmela-edited *Advanced Study of Gymnastics* is one of the best sources of current practice based upon physiological and medical research.

Foreign Literature

Fluency in German and French would go a long way towards providing the English-speaking teacher/coach with the broadest range of materials in gymnastics. The theoretical texts of the Russian coach Ukran are available in German as are several texts treating the biomechanics of gymnastics exclusively, the most recent of which is Söll's *Biomechanik in der Sportpraxis—Geräatturnen*. George's *Biomechanics for Women's Gymnastics* and an unpublished manuscript by Schmidt entitled *Scientific Approach to Women's Gymnastics* should help to clarify this sort of material for the English reader.

One of the better technical supplements for the field is *Der Turnwart* (published by Otto Pohl, Post Office Box 103, 31 Celle, Federal Republic of Germany), which is added monthly to *Deutsches Turnen*. The Japanese reader will also benefit from the highly technical *Japanese Journal of Gymnastics* (Hiro Okamura, 13–19 Nojima-Cho, Kanazawa-ku, Yokohama, Japan 236).

When materials from foreign publishing houses seem to be a desirable option, one of the best distributors of such materials in the United States is *Adler's Foreign Books, Inc.* (162 Fifth Ave., New York, N.Y., 10010). The Adler people have been most reliable in obtaining a number of titles from East Germany, Germany, and France. This service is prompt and efficient and eliminates confusion for those speaking and writing English only.

General Physical Education

Munrow's classic *Pure and Applied Gymnastics* remains the only text book that makes a strong theoretical case for gymnastics in the schools. Munrow examines a number of different approaches to gymnastics, providing an excellent set of references for theoretical issues. Mosston's *Teaching Physical Education* and *Developmental Movement* are both very good. The former has been used as an introduction to teaching methods and style in physical education with frequent reference to gymnastics. *The Magic of Gymnastics,* edited by George, is a compendium of material originally prepared for the Boston Convention of the American Association (now Alliance) for Health, Physical Education and Recreation. The Farkas *Age-Group Workbook* is still available from the USGF, but it has never been revised and is of limited value in club work. The *Workbook* is a good source of testing materials for the physical educator, however. Pedagogical materials of the French Gymnastic Federation (Rue Taitbout 15, 75009 Paris, France) provide excellent progression sequences. Almost every issue of *Education Physique et Sport* has one or more useful articles on gymnastic instruction which may be of value even to those whose French is somewhat limited (*EPS,* 11 Avenue de Tremblay, 75012 Paris, France). The only comparable resource in English would be the first twenty volumes of Sundby Publications, which are now available on microfilm. These volumes include all issues of *The Modern Gymnast, Gymnast,* and *International Gymnast* through 1976. More recent volumes are available on microfilm through University Microfilms in Ann Arbor, Michigan. Sundby Publications (410 Broadway, Santa Monica, Cal., 90401) has initiated the development of *International Gymnast's Technical Supplement* which should prove to be valuable in the physical education field. The *Supplement* is scheduled to be a quarterly.

Individual Events

There are few English-language books on individual gymnastic events. Most of these materials are available only through foreign publishers. The Kunzle series is still a unique source of information for individual events for men and boys, although the series is incomplete, lacking a volume for vaulting and rings. Kunzle's work is now a bit dated, but his suggestions for progression are sound. His four-volume resource is therefore a valuable addition to the gymnastic library.

The books listed below are thought to be among the best available. Foreign titles are generally available through Adler's Foreign Books, Inc. (See section on "Foreign Literature" above.) The books listed should be of value even for those who are restricted to English fluency.

Floor Exercise Kunzle's volume on *Free Standing* (Floor Exercise) contains some good suggestions for boys and men, while books listed below under "Tumbling" should also be helpful. Friesen's workbook on *Floor Exercise* is useful for the novice.

Vaulting No specialized books on vaulting have yet been developed in English. Basic vaulting techniques are given a thorough treatment in Koch's *Springen und Überschlagen—Hechten und Rollen,* which is one of a number of books in a paperback series produced by Karl Hoffman Publishers (Verlag Karl Hoffman, 7060 Schorndorf bei Stuttgart, Postf. 1360, Federal Republic of Germany), which publishes many specialized books on gymnastics. Taylor, Bajin, and Zivic have written a good chapter on vaulting in their *Olympic Gymnastics for Men & Women.*

Horizontal Bar In addition to Kunzle's volume on this subject, *La Barre Fixe* by Chautemps and Masino may be the best volume on the subject in the world. Its 632 pages are highly illustrated. The publisher, Vigot (23 Rue de l'Ecole de Médecine, 75006 Paris, France), has produced a number of excellent books including the well-known theoretical texts of Roland Carrasco.

Uneven Parallel Bars It is somewhat ironic that just prior to the "rediscovery" of gymnastics by Americans in 1960, the first specialty book of the modern period treating uneven bar work exclusively was published privately by Walter Lienert. The book was not republished or revised and went out-of-print. French authors Chautemps and Masino (see "Horizontal Bar" above) have produced a book on the unevens, and another by the well-known German coach Hans Timmermann is *Leistungsturnen am hohen Stufenbarren* in the Series previously noted published by Karl Hoffman. At the time of its first printing (1967) the American innovator, Doris Brause, was listed among the top internationals on this apparatus.

Balance Beam Koch and Timmermann have produced one specialty book on balance beam work (*Vom Steigen und Balancieren zum Turnen am Schwebebalken*) which is also published in the Hoffman Series.

Parallel Bars Kunzle's volume in the Olympic Gymnastic Series is the only specialty book in English.

Rings John Hinds' *Still Rings: Skills and Techniques* is a very helpful book and could become a model for other specialty publications in gymnastics.

Pommel Horse Kunzle's volume on pommel horse was published at a time when most Americans thought such a title sounded "funny." The book was very thoughtfully worked out and was then, as now, a valuable addition to the gymnastic library. Tonry's *The Side Horse* is a collection of photographic sequences which are useful in describing some of the more complicated movements on this apparatus.

Trampoline See Hennessy's article in this Manual.

Men and Boys

Hartley Price was the first author to contribute a book to the field in the modern era, and it was in use during World War II (*Gymnastics and Tumbling*). One of Price's students, Eric Hughes, has written one of the more successful books in this category (*Gymnastics for Men*), which utilizes a series of routines to acquaint the novice with a sequential learning plan. The routine approach is also utilized by Nik Stewart in his *Gymnastics for Men*, providing as many as twenty-four mini-routines in a graded progression. Stewart includes a training plan for conditioning and a training cycle to assist the gymnast in his preparation for competition. Ryser's *A Manual for Tumbling and Apparatus Stunts* is one of the best methods texts for teacher preparation. Now in its sixth edition, it is recommended by no less an authority than Gene Wettstone. Finally, Kaneko's *Olympic Gymnastics,* which has been translated for use in other countries, provides some insight into the training of boys and men in Japan. It is probably the best available book for use in gymnastic clubs. Tonry's *Gymnastics Illustrated* is an excellent source of illustrations for a majority of gymnastic movements for boys and men.

Miscellaneous Materials

Numerous gymnastic publications that touch upon related areas are both unique and valuable additions to the gymnastic library.

For example, Boone's *Better Gymnastics—How to Spot the Performer* is the only volume published to date that attempts to treat this very important topic exclusively. Although Boone has not provided a systematized or theoretical base for his work along the lines suggested by Vallière and Chouinard,[2] photographs illustrating experienced spotters at work provide some very practical knowledge for both men and women. Photographs of spotting action are also well done in Ito and Dolney's *Mastering Women's Gymnastics*.

Andrea Schmid's *Modern Rhythmic Gymnastics* is the best book available on the subject, and it has been translated for a French edition, a unique honor. Schmid has emerged as the most prominent American author in the field of women's gymnastics, having been primarily responsible for the development of the most widely used methods text for the field (*Gymnastics for Women*, with Drury), and she is a major contributor to *Judging and Coaching Women's Gymnastics* ("Uneven Parallel Bars"). Cumiskey's *Men's Judging Guide and Course* is published by the United States Gymnastic Federation (P.O. Box 12713, Tucson, Arizona, 85732). The USGF is also the source of all official publications of the International Gymnastic Federation (F.I.G.).

Among some of the unique items distributed by the USGF are the *Dictionary of Gymnastic Terminology* and Laptad's *History of the Development of the USGF*.

Rackham's *Diving Complete* is an excellent source of information on twisting, which has many gymnastic applications.

Judd's *Exhibition Gymnastics* is extremely helpful for those who plan periodic gymnastic exhibitions. This book draws on the years of experience of the highly successful Springfield College Exhibition Team.

A number of authors have attempted to write single volumes devoted to both the men's and women's programs. The most successful of these has been Loken and Willoughby's *The Complete Book of Gymnastics*, which in its third edition has been in use for twenty years.

Frederick's two paperback books in the Brown Physical Education Series (*Gymnastics for Women* and *Gymnastics for Men*) have seen wide use for more than a decade. The author introduces the method of thinking about gymnastics in terms of five families of movement. This concept will be expanded in a more comprehensive volume.

The best source of relatively inexpensive films on gymnastics is Frank Endo (12200 S. Berendo Ave., Los Angeles, Cal., 90044). Endo is also the U.S. distributor for a number of Japanese gymnastic books, many of which are highly illustrated. Loop films are available from the Athletic Institute (200 Castlewood Dr., North Palm Beach, Florida, 33408), which publishes a number of "Self Teaching" pamphlets for individual gymnastic events. The American Alliance for Health, Physical

2. Vallière, A. and Chouinard, J., "L'assistance manuelle en gymnastique sportive." *Mouvement* 3:109–125, 1968.

Education, Recreation and Dance (AAHPERD—1201 16th St., N.W., Washington, D.C., 20036) is another source of a number of loop films.

With an increased emphasis on equal opportunity for individuals with handicapping conditions, there is a need for materials that will help the teacher understand the special needs of such children and adults. Buchhalter's monograph (*Gymnastic Mainstreaming*) provides some initial insights for a variety of handicapping conditions as well as suggestions for appropriate gymnastic activity. Cratty's *Trampoline Activities for Atypical Children* provides evidence of the therapeutic value of this activity.

Tumbling

By 1979, all of the classic texts on tumbling had gone out of print. Three new books have appeared since 1977, none of which could compete with a revision of Szypula's *Tumbling and Balancing for All* were one available.[3]

The best treatment of tumbling fundamentals is found in Gabriel's *Tumbling and Balancing: Basic Skills and Variations*. The author presents a logical sequence of families of tumbling movements and good progressions. The most complete treatment of tumbling is Austin's *Winning Power Tumbling*. Intermediate and advanced movements are exposed by the author, who also includes highlights from the history of tumbling and an index to the current rules which have been adopted by the International Trampoline Federation. These rules should not be confused with those of the International Federation of Sports Acrobatics. There are special rules for acrotumbling, which employs a spring-enhanced floor. The United States Sports Acrobatics Federation is the source of the rules (P.O. Box 7, Santa Monica, California 90406).

Finally, Wiley's *The Tumbling Book* is the best source of information related to advanced performance.

Women and Girls

Schmid and Drury's *Gymnastics for Women,* now in its fourth edition, is the most complete source in the field. The range of information is inclusive of gymnastic dance, modern rhythmic gymnastics, and judging. Cooper's *Feminine Gymnastics,* in its third edition, is also an excellent source of realistic sequences of movement providing the gymnast with ideas for routine construction. *Mastering Women's Gymnastics* (Ito and Dolney) provides an up-to-date view of typical instruction in the gymnastic club. George's *Biomechanics of Women's Gymnastics* is a valuable source of technical information for both men and women.

The gymnastic program for girls and women has grown tremendously. This fact is reflected in the literature, with the appearance since 1960 of approximately twice as many books for females as males. Until the emergence of Kurt Thomas as a world class gymnast, no book was available in English describing the life and times of any prominent male gymnast, although a dozen or more have appeared for women.

---

3. The author might be able to supply copies of this book (George Szypula, Gymnastic Coach, Michigan State University, East Lansing, Michigan, 48823).

Conclusion

There is no question about the great potential for the future development of gymnastics in America. The point of producing the present Manual, which is itself a landmark development in the gymnastic literature, is the rational and safe conduct of all sorts of gymnastic programming.

The bulk of the current gymnastic literature is primarily clinical in nature. Accordingly, gymnastic wisdom is acquired by trial and error or learned through an apprenticeship. Standards for the measurement and certification of teachers and coaches have yet to be written, although the YMCA has developed some minimal criteria in its Progressive Gymnastics Program for Youth under the direction of W.P. Wortman.[4]

There are indications that theoretical concerns and a synthesis for the field are developing—the prime evidence for such a movement being found in an increasing number of manuscripts treating theoretical matters and the adaptation of theory to the demands of the clinician. Although it would be difficult to identify any single volume as *the* definitive work in gymnastics, the status of our literature is very healthy and is growing.

---

4. Wortman, W.P., Editor, *National YMCA Progressive Gymnastics Program for Youth.* New York: National YMCA Program Materials (291 Broadway, New York, N.Y., 10017), 1978.

Selected Bibliography

AAHPER Position Statements on Trampolines, *Journal of Physical Education and Recreation,* October, 1978.

AAHPERD (American Alliance for Health, Physical Education, Recreation and Dance), 1201 16th St., N.W., Washington, D.C., 20036—Source of loop films for gymnastics.

Aaron, G.S., *The Science of Trampolining.* Cardiff CF2 6HT, Great Britain: John Jones Cardiff Ltd., 1970.

ASTM (American Society for Testing and Materials), Standard Consumer Safety Specification for Components, Assembly, and Use of a Trampoline. 1916 Race St., Philadelphia 19103, reprinted annually.

Athletic Institute, 200 Castlewood Dr., North Palm Beach, Florida, 33408—Source of loop films for gymnastics.

Austin, Jeff, *Winning Power Tumbling.* Chicago: Contemporary Books, 1978.

————, *Winning Trampoline.* Chicago: Contemporary Books, 1976

Aziz, J.A., *How to Teach Gymnastics—Tumbling and Balancing.* The author, 551 Chiddington Ave., London, Ontario, Canada.

Boone, Wm. T., *Better Gymnastics—How to Spot the Performer.* Mountain View, Cal.: World Publications, Inc., 1978.

Bowers, Carolyn (with Fie, Kjeldsen and Schmid), *Judging and Coaching Women's Gymnastics.* Palo Alto, Cal.: Mayfield Publishers, 1972.

Braecklein, Heinz, *Trampolinturnen II.* Frankfurt, Germany: Wilhelm Limpert Publishers, 1974.

Brown, Margaret and Sommer, Betty, *Movement Education: Its Evolution and a Modern Approach.* Reading, Mass.: Addison-Wesley, 1969.

Buchhalter, Adrian, *Gymnastic Mainstreaming.* Graduate Synthesis Project, State University College at Brockport, Brockport, N.Y., 14420, 1979.

Chautemps, G. and Masino, P., *La Barre Fixe.* Paris: Vigot Publishers, 1961.

————, *Les Barres à Hauteurs Inégales.* Paris: Vigot Publishers, n.d.

Cochrane, Tuovi, *International Gymnastics for Girls and Women.* Reading, Mass.: Addison-Wesley, 1969.

Cooper, Phyllis, *Feminine Gymnastics.* (3rd Ed.) Minneapolis: Burgess Publishing Co., 1979.

Cratty, B.J., *Trampoline Activities for Atypical Children.* Mountain View, Cal.: Peek Publications, 1969.

Cumiskey, Frank, *Men's Judging Guide and Course.* Tucson: USGF, 1977.

Diem, Liselott, *Children Learn Physical Skills* (Vol. 1, Birth to 3 Years; Vol. 2, 4–6 Years), Distributed by AAHPERD in cooperation with the German copyright holder, Kosel Publishers of Munich, 1974.

Endo, Frank, U.S. distributor for current Japanese gymnastic texts and the source of inexpensive films for all major international gymnastic competitions. 12200 S. Berendo Ave., Los Angeles, 90044.

Farkas, James, *Age Group Gymnastic Workbook*. Tucson: USGF, n.d.

Frederick, A.B., *Gymnastics for Women*. Dubuque, Iowa: Wm. C. Brown Co., 1966.

————, *Gymnastics for Men*. Dubuque, Iowa: Wm. C. Brown Co., 1969.

Friesen, Jo, *Floor Exercise—Student Workbook*. Lafayette, Indiana: Balt Publishers, 1974.

Gabriel, Judith, *Tumbling and Balancing—Basic Skills and Variations*. Englewood Cliffs, N.J.: Prentice-Hall, Inc., 1977.

George, Gerald, Editor, *The Magic of Gymnastics*. Santa Monica, Cal.: Sundby Publications, 1970.

————, *Biomechanics of Women's Gymnastics*. Englewood Cliffs, N.J.: Prentice-Hall Inc., 1979.

Griswold, Larry and Wilson, Glenn, *Trampoline Tumbling Today*. Cranbury, N.J.: A.S. Barnes and Co., Inc., 1969.

Harris, Rich, *The Trampoline for Physical Education—Instructor's Edition*. San Mateo, Cal.: The Pea Press, 1977.

Hennessy, Jeff T., *Trampolining*. Dubuque, Iowa: Wm. C. Brown Co., 1968.

————, *The Trampoline As I See It*. (2nd Ed.) Lafayette, Louisiana: International Publications, 1969.

Hughes, Eric, Editor, *Gymnastics for Girls*. (2nd Ed.) New York: Wiley, 1971.

————, *Gymnastics for Men*. New York: Wiley, 1966.

Ito, Robert and Dolney, Pam C., *Mastering Women's Gymnastics*. Chicago: Contemporary Books, Inc., 1978.

Judd, Leslie, et al., *Exhibition Gymnastics*. New York: Association Press, 1969.

Kaneko, Akimoto, *Olympic Gymnastics*. New York: Sterling Publishing Co., Inc., 1976.

Kjeldsen, Kitty, *Women's Gymnastics*. (2nd Ed.) Boston: Allyn and Bacon, 1975.

Koch, Karl, *Springen und Überschlagen—Hechten und Rollen*. (Practice of Physical Education Series-#2) Schorndorf, W. Germany: Karl Hoffmann Publisher, 1965.

Koch, Karl and Timmerman, H., *Vom Steigen und Balancieren zum Turnen am Schwebebalken*. (Practice of Physical Education Series-#5) Schorndorf, W. Germany: Karl Hoffmann Publisher, 1973.

Kunzle, George, *Olympic Gymnastics—Horizontal Bar*. London: Barrie and Rockliff, 1957.

————, *Olympic Gymnastics—Pommel Horse*. London: Barrie and Rockliff, 1960.

————, *Olympic Gymnastics—Parallel Bars*. London: Barrie and Rockliff, 1966.

Kunzle, George and Thomas, B.W., *Olympic Gymnastics—Free Standing*. (Floor Exercise) London: Barrie and Rockliff, 1956.

Laptad, Richard, *History and Development of the United States Gymnastic Federation*. Tucson: USGF, 1972.

Loken, Newt and Willoughby, Robert, *Complete Book of Gymnastics*. (3rd Ed.) Englewood Cliffs, N.J.: Prentice-Hall, Inc., 1977.

Mauldon, E. and Layson, J., *Teaching Gymnastics and Body Control*. (Themes for Movement Education etc.) Boston: Plays, Inc., 1965.

Mosston, Muska, *Developmental Movement*. Columbus, Ohio: C.E. Merrill, 1965.

————, *Teaching Physical Education*. Columbus, Ohio: C.E. Merrill, 1966.

Munrow, A.D., *Pure and Applied Gymnastics*. (2nd Ed.) London: Edward Arnold, Ltd., 1963.

NAGWS Gymnastic Guide. Published periodically by AAHPERD. (See AAHPERD entry for address.)

O'Quinn, Garland, *Gymnastics for Elementary School Children.* Manchaca, Texas: Sterling Swift, 1973.

Price, Hartley, et al., *Gymnastics and Tumbling.* New York: Arco Publishing Co., Inc., 1972.

Ryser, Otto, *Manual for Tumbling and Apparatus Stunts.* (6th Ed.) Dubuque, Iowa: Wm. C. Brown, 1976.

Salmela, John, Ed., *The Advanced Study of Gymnastics.* Springfield, Ill.: C.C. Thomas, 1976.

Schmid, Andrea, *Modern Rhythmic Gymnastics.* Palo Alto, Cal.: Mayfield Publishing Co., 1976.

Schmid, Andrea and Drury, Blanche J., *Gymnastics for Women.* (4th Ed.) Palo Alto, Cal.: Mayfield Publishing Co., 1977.

Schulz, Dieter, *Methodik des Trampolinspringens.* (Practice of Physical Education Series - #52) Schorndorf, W. Germany: Karl Hoffmann Publisher, 1972.

Söll, Hans, *Biomechanik in der Sportpraxis—Gerätturnen.* (Practice of Physical Education Series - #96) Schorndorf, W. Germany: Karl Hoffman, Publisher, 1975.

Straus, Hal, Ed., *The Gymnastics Guide.* Mountain View, Cal.: World Publications, 1978.

Stuart, Nik, *Gymnastics for Men.* London: Stanley Paul, 1978. (U.S. Distributor is Hutchinson Publishing Inc., 99 Main St., Salem, New Hampshire, 03079)

Szypula, George, *Tumbling and Balancing for All.* The author, Michigan State University, East Lansing, Mich. 48823.

Tatlow, Peter, et al., *The World of Gymnastics.* New York: Atheneum Publishers, 1978.

Taylor, Bryce, Bajin, B. and Zivic, T., *Olympic Gymnastics for Men and Women.* Englewood Cliffs, N.J.: Prentice-Hall, Inc., 1972.

Timmermann, Hans, *Leistungsturnen am Hohen Stufenbarren.* (Practice of Physical Education Series - #17) Schorndorf, W. Germany: Karl Hoffmann Publisher, 1967.

Tonry, Don, *The Side Horse.* Northbridge, Mass.: Gymnastic Aids, n.d.

———, *Gymnastics Illustrated.* Northbridge, Mass.: Gymnastic Aids, 1972.

Ukran, M.L., *Gerätturnen.* (Translated from Russian to German by Heinz Neumann and Karl-Heinz Zschocke.) Berlin, GDR: Sportverlag Berlin, 1976.

———, *Technik der Turnubungen.* (Translated to German from Russian by Peter Braun) Berlin, GDR: Sportverlag Berlin, 1970.

United States Gymnastic Federation (USGF) P.O. Box 12713, Tucson, Arizona, 85711.

Wachtel, Erna and Loken, Newt, *Girls' Gymnastics.* New York: Sterling Publishing Co., Inc., 1967.

Weaver, Ernestine R., *Gymnastics for Girls and Women.* Englewood Cliffs, N.J.: Prentice-Hall, Inc., 1968.

Wiley, Jack, *The Tumbling Book.* New York: David McKay Co., Inc., 1977.

Wortman, W. Philip, Ed., *National YMCA Progressive Gymnastics Program for Youth.* National YMCA Program Materials (291 Broadway, New York, N.Y., 10017), 1978.

Contributors

NORMAN BARNES, Advertising Director, Nissen Corporation; former Big Ten Tennis Champion, University of Iowa

ROBERT J. BEVENOUR, President, Nissen Corporation

CAP CAUDILL, President, Louisville School of Gymnastics; member, National Elite Development Committee for Women; board member, USGSA

ROY DAVIS, Director and Owner, Gymnastics West, Palo Alto, CA; Team Captain, University of California, Berkeley, 1960; studied in Japan 1966–69

THOMAS L. DUNN, Jr., College of Health, Physical Education, and Recreation, Penn State University; Assistant Gymnastic Coach; Vice President N.G.C.A.; NCAA Co-Champion, 1971

STORMY EATON, The Desert Gymnastic Training Center USA, Tempe, AZ; NCAA F. E. Champion, 1971; 2nd World Tumbling Championships, 1974

DAVID A. FEIGLEY, Ph.D., Assistant Professor, Psychology, Rutgers University; Director of the Feigley School of Gymnastics

LARRY FIE, President, AMF American Athletic Equipment Division

A. B. FREDERICK, Ph.D., Professor and Gymnastic Coach, State University College at Brockport, New York; author of gymnastics texts

JAY GEIST, Field Representative, Nissen Corporation; gymnastic team, Temple University

ABIE GROSSFELD, Professor and Gymnastic Coach, Southern Connecticut State College, New Haven; NCAA Champion, 1958; Olympic Coach, 1972; Olympian, 1956, Coach of the Year; NCAA Team Championships author of gymnastics texts

JEFF T. HENNESSY, Associate Professor and Trampoline Coach, University of Southwestern Louisiana; Technical Chairman of FIT, AAU; USA World Trampoline Team Coach or Judge, 1964–78; author of trampoline texts

ERIC HUGHES, Ph.D., Professor and Gymnastic Coach, University of Washington, Seattle; author of two textbooks on competitive gymnastics for men and women

LOYD J. HUVAL, Instructor in Gymnastics, University of New Orleans; author of two textbooks on gymnastics

EDMUND ISABELLE, Director of Woodward Gymnastic Camp; former Assistant Coach at Penn State University; NCAA Championship team, 1965

MIKE JACKI, Director of Promotions, AMF American Athletic Equipment Division; Director of Camp Tsukara, Wisconsin; four times Big 8 Conference Champion, Iowa State University; NCAA Champion and All-American

ALEXANDER KALENAK, M.D., Division of Orthopedic Surgery, Hershey Medical Center, The Pennsylvania State University; Orthopedic Surgeon for the Penn State Athletic Department

EDGAR M. KNEPPER, Executive Director, U.S. Association of Independent Gymnastic Clubs; Director of Olympiad Schools, Wilmington, DEL.

HAYES KRUGER, Assistant Professor of Physical and Health Education and Gymnastic Coach, Madison College, Harrisonburg, VA; author of text on movement education in physical education

CAROLE LIEDTKE, Associate Professor in Physical Education and Gymnastic Coach, University of Louisville; international judge

DAVID J. LINDSTROM, Coordinator for Emergency Care Education, Penn State University; author of National Standards Paramedic Curriculum; member of National Academy of Science/National Research Council

NEWTON C. LOKEN, Ed.D., Associate Professor and Gymnastic Coach, University of Michigan; 12 Big Ten Team Championships; author of gymnastic texts; NCAA Team Champions, 1963–70

RUTH ANN McBRIDE, Director, MarVa Teens; board member, USGSA

RODI NIKITINS, Director of Nikitins School of Dance and Gymnastics, Seattle; professional acrobat, "Flying Rinaldos"; USO Shows; Swan Lake Ballet

KARL SCHWENZFEIER, Lt. Colonel, Air Force, Retired; Director of Gymnastics, Penn State; Olympian, 1956; USA Olympic Coach, 1976; NCAA, NAAU Champion, 1956

GARY R. SEIBERT, President, Gym-Kin, Inc.; board member, USGSA

ROBERT STOUT, Teacher of Health and Physical Education at Abington High School; Technical Director of the N.G.J.A. (east); Olympian, 1952; NCAA Champion, 1949; NAAU All-Around Champion, 1952–53

WILLIAM G. STRAUSS, Director of Parkette Gymnastic Club; National Elite Women's Development Director, 1976; USA women's coach, Moscow News Championships

GEORGE SZYPULA, Associate Professor of Physical Education and Gymnastic Coach, Michigan State University; author of gymnastic texts; NCAA Champion, 1942, 1958; NAAU Tumbling Champ, 1942–43

DONALD R. TONRY, Instructor in Physical Education and Gymnastic Coach, Yale University; author of many texts; Olympian, 1960; NCAA Champion, 1956–59

ZAHIR TOBY TOWSON, Artistic Director, Musawwir Gymnastic Dance Company, New York; 6 times National F.E. Champion; NCAA Champion, 1968–69

BETTY VAN DER SMISSEN, J.D., Ph.D.; Member of the Kansas Bar; Director, School of Health, Physical Education and Recreation, Bowling Green State University

GREGOR WEISS, Associate Professor of Business, Prince George's College, Washington, D.C.; Director of the GM School of Gymnastics; Olympian, 1964; NCAA and Pan Am Champion, 1961, 1962